# Unleashing the Right Side of the Brain

# Unleashing the Right Side of the Brain

## The LARC Creativity Program

Robert H. Williams, Ph.D.
and
John Stockmyer

THE STEPHEN GREENE PRESS
Lexington, Massachusetts

First published in 1987 by The Stephen Greene Press, Inc.
Published simultaneously in Canada by Penguin Books Canada Limited
Distributed by Viking Penguin Inc., 40 West 23rd Street, New York, NY 10010.

Cartoons by Sam Michael Cangelosi
Line drawings by John Stockmyer

**Library of Congress Cataloging-in-Publication Data**
Williams, Robert H. (Robert Howard)
Unleashing the right side of the brain.
Bibliography
1. Creative thinking. 2. Cerebral dominance.
I. Stockmyer, John. II. Title. III. Title: LARC
creativity program.
BF408.W53 1987 153.3'5 87-187
ISBN 0-8289-0620-3

Designed by Denise Hoffman
Printed in the United States of America
by The Alpine Press, Inc.
Set in Clearface and Dom Casual Diagonal by WordTech
Produced by Unicorn Production Services

*I'd like to dedicate this book to my parents, Earl and Mary Williams, who gave me all the love they had and all the opportunities they never had.*

—Robert H. Williams

*I dedicate this book to me, first for picking loving parents, then for having the good sense to marry a lady named Connie.*

—John Stockmyer

# Contents

# Preface

Readers interested in the research and methodology that supports LARC (Left And Right Creativity) may wish to consult the following studies:

> "The Left and Right of Creativity: A Cognitive (Hemispheric Cooperation) Based Program for Teaching Creative Thinking," by Robert H. Williams, John Stockmyer, and Sharon Ann Williams (*The Creative Child and Adult Quarterly,* Vol. IX, No. 2, 1984).
>
> "A Comparative Study of the Effectiveness of the Williams-Stockmyer Creativity System in Promoting the Creative Thinking of Sixth Grade Children." Nancy C. Stovall and Robert H. Williams (*The Creative Child and Adult Quarterly,* Vol. X, No. 2, 1985).

The listing of the authors is arbitrary, denoting equal contribution to the ideas, research, and preparation of the work.

# Acknowledgments

Since nothing happens in a vacuum, it is no surprise that this book could not have been written without the intellectual input and great good will of my colleagues at Maple Woods Community College (part of the Metropolitan Community College system of Kansas City Missouri). Maple Woods puts into practice the principles of freedom, originality, concern, and excellence, these qualities providing a rich atmosphere in which *many* "good things" happen to students, faculty, staff, and administration — and to the community at large.

— John Stockmyer

I agree with John. Maple Woods is a great place to teach and a great place to be. I have just started my teaching career at Maple Woods, but my connection to the school began when I was a member of its first graduating class. Since that time, I have attended five different colleges and universities. Many of these have provided fine experiences, but by far the best teaching I have ever received was at Maple Woods. Maple Woods continues to be a home for academic freedom and educational excellence. It is a *true* campus of achievement!

— Robert H. Williams

# Introduction

*Create:* "To produce . . . along new or unconventional lines. . . . To make or bring into existence something new."
— *Webster's Third New International Dictionary*

How often have you heard someone say, "I wish I could be a creative person like so-and-so"? Many of us *do* long to be more creative but are discouraged about our chances to become so because we believe that inventive people have inherited their imaginative powers as surely as the high school beauty queen was born with good skin, glistening teeth, and baby blue eyes. Most people have always assumed that the mysterious process called creativity is a supernatural gift granted only to a chosen few and that you and I can do nothing but envy the da Vincis, the Beethovens, and the Edisons of this world who are foreordained to receive the rewards society reserves for those who can generate imaginative ideas. But is it really true that a few people just *are* creative? Fresh insights are rare and do seem to come to some people out of "nowhere," but . . .

A few years ago, Robert Williams (a psychologist and designer of simulation games) began to discover ways for tapping human inventiveness. Long interested in creativity—and operating from a broad educational background (in addition to a Ph.D., he holds three master's degrees)—Dr. Williams invented a system for producing the special kind of left-right brain switches that seem to be responsible for the formation of new ideas.

In the process of developing his Creativity Program, Williams began a collaboration with John Stockmyer, a friend and history professor with a long record of creative accomplishments. Winner of several teaching awards, Professor Stockmyer's instruction is marked by innovative approaches, including the building of a time-machine simulator with which to give his students "direct" experience of the past. An educational writer of dramatic records and filmstrips as well as a produced playwright, Stockmyer became the primary writer of the team, using his talents as a teacher to simplify and to explain Williams's ideas about creativity. Together, they began five years of investigations into the refinement and uses of LARC (*L*eft *A*nd *R*ight *C*reativity)—a step-by-step guide for anyone wishing to increase his or her originality.

The purpose of this book is to take you along a truly fascinating journey toward unlocking the mystery of the imaginative process, then to an understanding of the latest scientific findings about the bizarre workings of the human brain, and finally, through LARC, which serves as a personal guide through the labyrinth of the imaginative side of the human mind. In short, whether you are "naturally inventive" or anything but, this book can help you become more creative. Yes, even you!

# *Unleashing the Right Side of the Brain*

# part I
# About Creativity

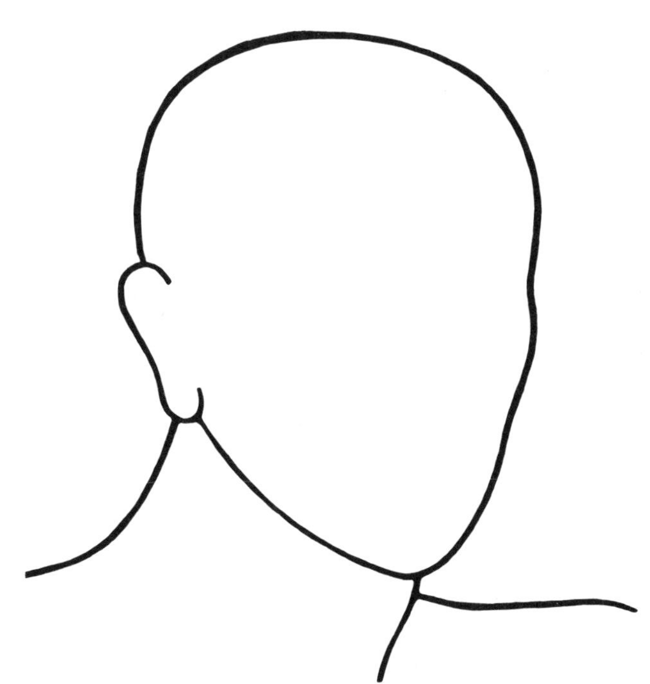

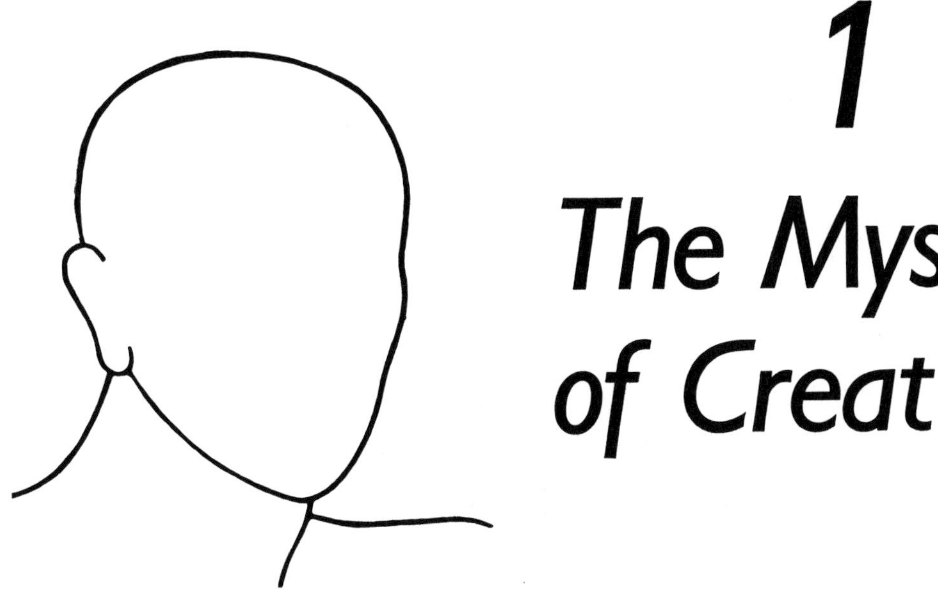

# 1 The Mystery of Creativity

## The Right Brain and Creativity

"How extremely stupid not to have thought of that" was the comment of the biologist Thomas Huxley upon first hearing about Darwin's new theory of evolution. By calling himself "stupid," Huxley could not have meant that he lacked mental capacity, for he was a scientist of extraordinary renown. It was just that, possessing many of the same "facts" about biology available to Darwin, Huxley had not used this information to come up with the novel idea of evolution. And so he *felt* stupid. This Huxley-Darwin illustration points out a truth that is sometimes overlooked: a person's *intellectual* abilities and *creative* prowess are not the same thing at all. (Another example of this dissimilarity is the observation that, though a high school student may *understand* calculus, it takes the imaginative genius of a Newton or a Leibnitz to *invent* calculus.)

We all know how to improve our knowledge, our grasp of the "facts," of course. We do this by reading, going to school, conversing with informed acquaintances. But what can be done to increase the inventive abilities of those of us who feel "stupid" when we discover that others always seem to be the ones who get the good ideas? Not much . . . until now. Past efforts to improve creativity have largely been generalized suggestions. Interesting. Inspirational. But hardly the systemized, nuts-and-bolts program most people need to become more inventive.

That no specific system has been discovered to prompt the imaginative side of the human personality is not for want of trying, of course, attempts having long been made to strengthen people's creativity or mental abilities in general — sometimes with amusing results. In the early 1800s, for instance, "scientists" called phrenologists decided that a person's intellect and character could be read in the bumps on his head, lumps that had been caused by "mental muscles" building up under the skull. Phrenologists even suggested that some people could benefit from sleeping on special pillows or wearing certain hats that would force the development of head bumps in other, more "productive" areas of the skull.

In more modern times, scientists have done a number of serious studies of inventive people, in an attempt to unlock the "secrets" of the so-called naturally creative. Unfortunately, even *these* investigations have uncovered little that could help the rest of us generate those all-important breakthrough ideas.

First made skeptical by earlier, "wild" efforts to enhance imagination, then disappointed that modern science has not produced techniques to stimulate inventiveness, many people have given up, believing that creativity just can't be taught. But it *can*, and that is precisely the purpose of this book—to teach creativity, something that our research on the right brain has shown can now be done!

## The Right Brain "Unleashed"

For some time, there has been good evidence to support the theory that the right side of the human brain is especially skilled at creative thinking. But since most people's right brains are so completely dominated by their logical, unimaginative left brains, this knowledge of right brain function has done little good. Then, some years ago, investigations by the authors began to suggest techniques that would "unleash" the right brain so that its creative input could break through the left brain's defenses. Additional experimentation produced a system in which *both* brains would work cooperatively to produce new and sensible solutions to almost any problem a person wished to explore. In this book, we present this system in a step-by-step creativity program called LARC: *L*eft *A*nd *R*ight *C*reativity.

## LARC

LARC (*L*eft *A*nd *R*ight *C*reativity) is a systematic approach to unlocking every person's imaginative potential. Given here in four versions—LARC I through IV—LARC will help the reader gain imaginative insight into practically any creativity problem. LARC stimulates the right brain while, at the same time, bringing the left brain into play; both brain halves are necessary for the fullest development of the creative process.

## What to Expect

Part I of the book provides useful background information about creativity, plus an overview of the latest scientific findings about the inventive nature of the brain. In Part II, LARC is taught in its four forms—LARC I and LARC II designed for relatively simple creativity problems and LARC III and IV suggested for more complex questions. Finally, Part III of the book cites a number of examples of how

LARC can be used in real life, how it might help someone find a solution for problems in academic matters, self-understanding, work-related issues, or personal relationships.

## What Is Creativity?

Creativity is the ability to imagine or invent something new. The truly inventive idea often seems to come from nowhere in a rare flash of insight that startles the creator as much as it does the rest of us. What is the origin of these mysterious, original concepts? How did the great thinkers — Galileo, Newton, Einstein — the practical men of genius — Bell, Edison, Ford — or the literary and artistic titans — Shakespeare and Picasso — generate their novel ideas? For that matter, how did Aunt Flossie come up with her special recipe for cinnamon-vinegar brownies? Unfortunately, creative people, both of the past and present, have great difficulty explaining how they form their inspired ideas. They may discuss the line of thought they were following at the time or point out the background knowledge without which they could not have discovered their novel ideas. They may be able to describe in detail the precise moment, even the exact place they were standing in the street when that GREAT IDEA flashed into their minds. But when it comes to explaining how the revolutionary concept was generated, they slide off into such phrases as, "It just popped into my mind." or "I was driving down the street when, all of a sudden, it dawned on me that . . ." Imaginative people have no more idea than the average person about how to churn up creative insights.

A young man related just such a "driving down the street" experience. "I was driving in heavy, downtown traffic when, somehow, I got this great idea for a couple of lines of a poem that I could write for my girl friend. I was afraid I would forget them — since I don't get these inspirations very often — so I pulled to the side of the street to write them down. Unfortunately, what with the city traffic and all, I still stopped other cars for about a minute while I wrote stuff down. But I had to do it because I didn't know if I would ever think of those words again." (It should be

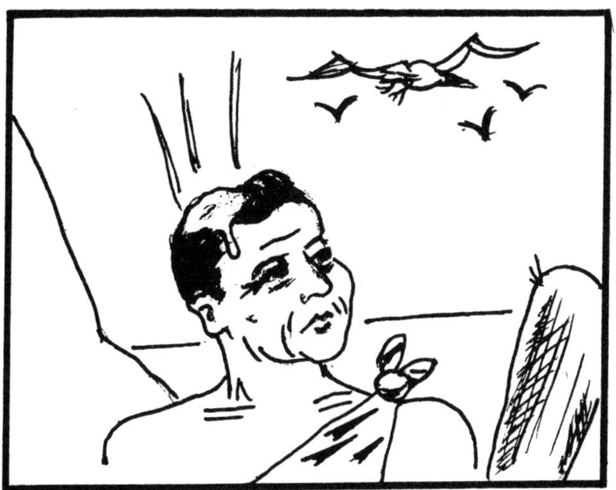

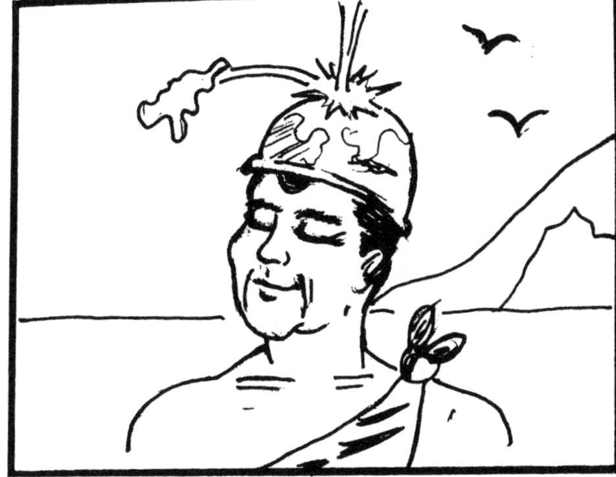

*Strategic Defense Initiative in the Stone Age.*

added that since the young man in question was built like a blockhouse the other motorists proved especially courteous in granting him time to record his poetic inspiration.)

That fresh ideas seem to come "out of the blue," suddenly, unexpectedly, is a common experience throughout history, though different ages have offered widely differing explanations about the sources of inventive visions. Since modern ideas about creativity have developed from earlier beliefs, a quick, historical review of what our ancestors thought about the origins of the inventive spark follows. And where better to start such a review than with the ancient Greeks, known for their inventiveness in politics (they created democracy), philosophy, drama, and architecture.

## *Greek Concepts of Creativity*

Twenty-five hundred years ago, Greeks believed they lived in a god-saturated universe, every rock and spring and mountain guarded by its nature spirit. They thought the inspiration for originality came from the gods and even invented heavenly creatures — the Muses — as supervisors of human creativity. The philosopher Socrates describes the imaginative process:

> . . . for a poet is a light and winged thing, and holy and never able to compose until he has become inspired, and is beside himself, and reason is no longer in him. . . . for not by art do they utter these, but by power divine. . . . Herein lies the reason why the deity has bereft them of their senses, and uses them as ministers, along with soothsayers and godly seers; it is in order that we listeners may know that it is not they who utter these precious revelations while their mind is not within them, but that it is god himself who speaks, and through them becomes articulate to us.

In this passage, Socrates presents standard Greek concepts that relate to the creative process: inspired thoughts originate with the gods, ideas coming not when a person is rational, but when someone is "beside himself," when "bereft" of his senses. Since the gods take away reason before bestowing the gift of inspiration, "thinking" might actually prevent the reception of divinely inspired revelations. Working on the assumption that the human mind might block out godly whisperings, Greek priests and prophets often suppressed their reason by chewing laurel leaves or taking opium. The faithful would also put themselves into a "mindless" state by mumbling chants or performing rhythmic dances to produce a kind of hypnotic numbing of their intellect, for it was in those trancelike, often manic moments that the human personality was thought to be most receptive to inspiration from above. One god, Apollo, was said to speak through a priestess, only after she had been drugged by breathing natural gas that hissed through a crack in the earth beneath her. Aesculapius, the god of healing, was supposed to reveal cures by visiting drugged patients in their dreams.

Even after later Greek philosophers and scientists turned away from strictly

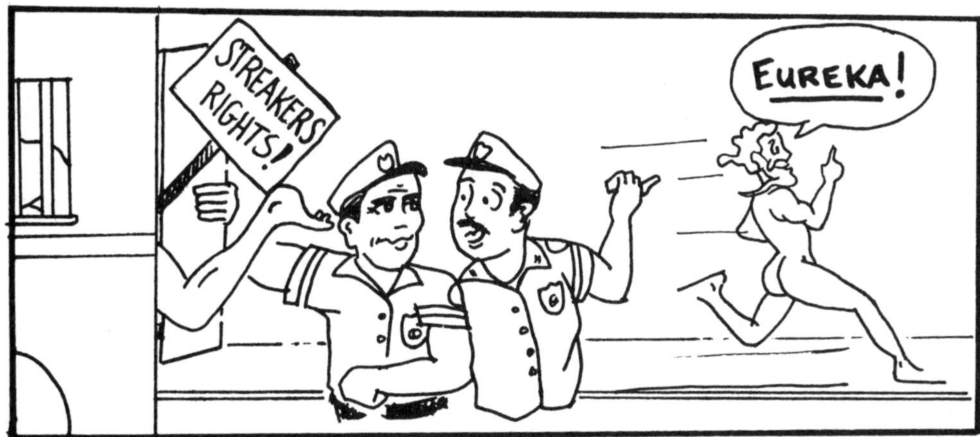

*"He's O.K. He's working on the problem of specific gravity of materials."*

religious explanations for unusual happenings, creative revelations still seemed random and unexplainable. The most famous example of the unpredictability of fresh ideas is the reported experience of the Greek physicist, Archimedes of Syracuse. Archimedes had been working on the problem of Hieron's crown (an experiment that does not concern us here). Failing to find the solution, Archimedes later discovered the answer while lowering himself into his bath. Noticing that his body's submersion caused the waterline on the side of the tub to rise, he suddenly had the riddle's answer. The thought so excited him that he forgot to dress and ran naked through the street toward his laboratory. "Eureka!" he shouted (I've found it!). Archimedes discovered a way to measure the specific gravity of materials, but certainly not by following a rational, step-by-step process. The answer just came to him suddenly, when he least expected it.

With the fall of the Roman Empire, the ancient world came to an end, to be followed by the Middle Ages, a thousand-year period that offered nothing new on the source of creativity. In fact, in the religiously inflexible atmosphere of medieval Europe, it was believed that inspiration could come as readily from the devil and his minions as from God and his angels, a concept that made *any* new idea suspect.

## The Nineteenth Century

In the modern world, people have increasingly begun to feel that creative ideas come not from "beyond" but rather from "within" — from some hidden part of the mind.

By the beginning of the nineteenth century, men were referring to this secret part of the brain as man's "inner Africa," like the yet-to-be-explored Dark Continent itself, a place of danger but also of promise. But how could a person tap this mysterious mental land, the very source of fruitful visions? Since the rational, reasonable side of human nature did not seem to produce original thoughts, it was hoped that the *emotional* side of man might be the key to imaginative inspiration.

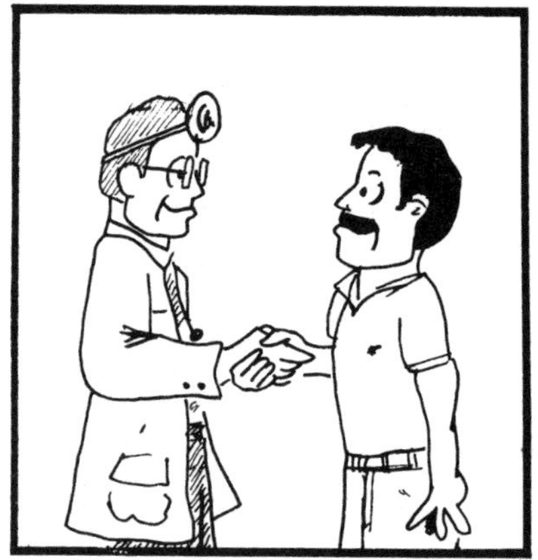

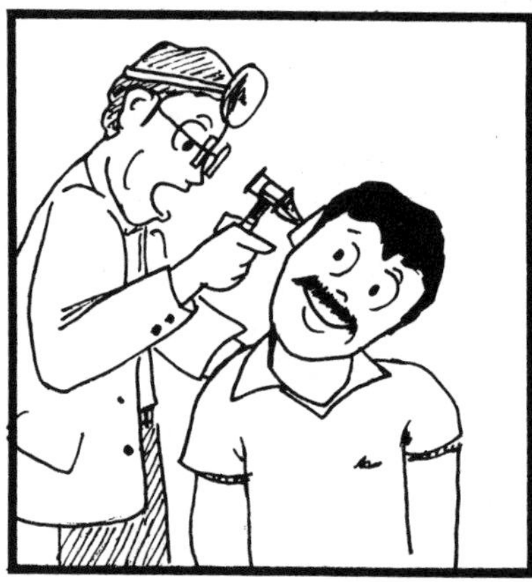

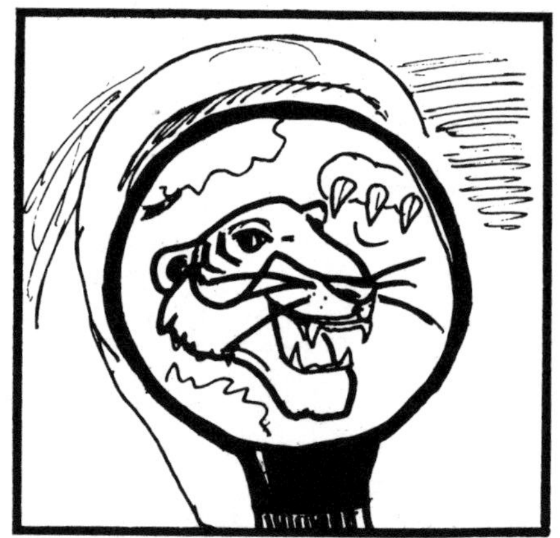

Because some individuals thought the strict social constraints of the last century stifled the emotionally stimulating experiences necessary to creativity, they tried to court new ideas by becoming passionate, unconventional, even rebellious. In this vein, famous poets of the early nineteenth century come to mind, in particular, Percy Shelley and his friend Lord Byron. Shelley's atheism (which prevented him from gaining custody of two of his children) and his depth of passion (including his attempted suicide) fit the pattern of the creative poets of his day. Lord Byron led an even more tempestuous life. Byron's love affairs were legion (the most famous, an incestuous relationship with his half sister) — his house in Italy filled, reported Shelley, with "caged wild animals and uncaged mistresses."

In fact, creativity *is* often linked with the "unusual" life. Take the case of the famous, late nineteenth-century scientist, Sir Francis Galton. A cousin of Darwin's with an estimated IQ of 200, Galton was interested in all sorts of things — making glasses for divers and doing studies on everything from Australian marriage customs, gregariousness in cattle, and rabbit breeding to the speed of trotting

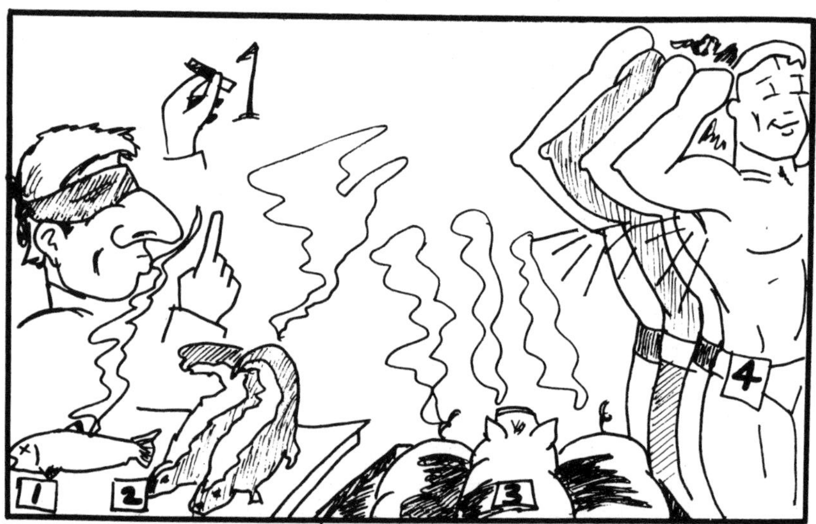

horses and (our favorite) arithmetic by smell. He invented the Galton whistle, which emits a pitch too high to be heard by the human ear. No doubt some men of his day questioned the value of having a whistle that *couldn't be heard,* though the silent dog whistle is one practical offshoot of that invention. Another time, wishing to know what it felt like to worship an idol, he began concentrating on a picture of Punch (a popular cartoon character), trying to feel reverence for it. The experiment worked; Galton developed special affection for that image. Can you imagine what someone else would have thought on learning that Galton was trying to worship a picture? But Galton didn't care; he was interested only in proving something about human nature — that just by a concentration of time and affection, you can love practically anything (which, now that you think about it, is why you care so much for your cat, car, children, and spouse!).

Another strange experiment undertaken by this unconventional man was when he wanted to discover what it felt like to become insane. To accomplish this, he began walking about the city, trying to imagine that every person, animal, and "thing" was spying on him. At first this didn't work, but gradually he began to feel it was really true. Galton even began to notice that there were horses that were obviously attempting to disguise their identity as spies by pretending to *pay no attention to him at all.* But is this really possible? Can people work themselves into paranoid states just by thinking themselves in jeopardy? (Remember the time when you came home alone from the midnight horror show and began to pay special attention to all those scary noises in the house? Hmm.) Galton's "insane" experiment helped in the understanding of human behavior, but it is related here to highlight the man's courage in performing what others would call laughable experiments, not letting himself be intimidated by what THEY might think. (In case even you are tempted to dismiss Galton as just another English eccentric, consider that he was presented with a gold medal for his explorations in Africa, elected a Fellow of the Royal Society, and knighted in 1909.)

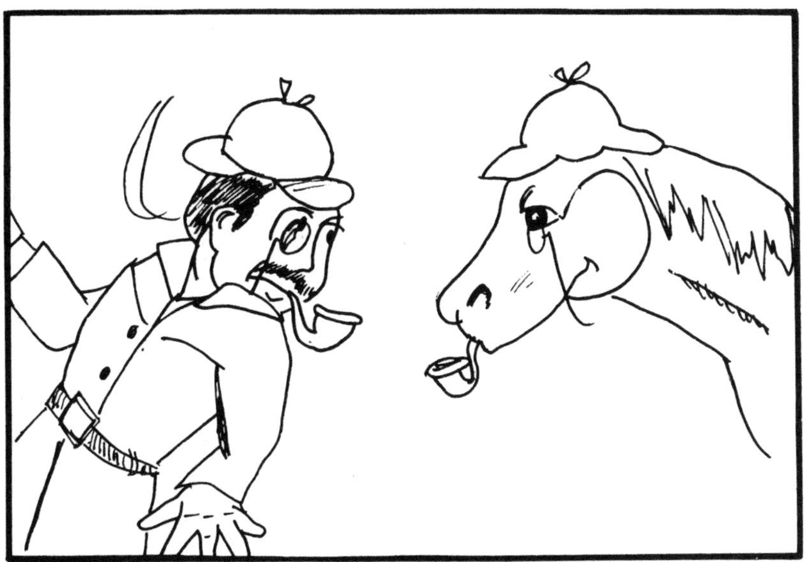

## *To Sleep: Perchance to . . .*

As we have seen, some have believed that living an unusual life style aided the creative process. But how does this fit with the experience of the poet Coleridge who said he composed an entire poem, not as a result of some emotionally liberating outburst, but *in his sleep*? Awaking, he had only to write:

> *In Xanadu did Kubla Khan a stately pleasure-dome decree:*
> *Where Alph, the sacred river, ran through caverns*
> *Measureless to man, down to a sunless sea.*

After jotting down several more stanzas, Coleridge was interrupted by a messenger and returned to the poem to discover that it, like the dream that produced it, had dissolved, never to appear to him again. Nor is Coleridge unique in having inspirational dreams. The nineteenth-century chemist F. A. Kekulé reported that his studies:

> . . . did not go well . . . I turned the chair to the fireplace and sank into a half sleep. The atoms flitted before my eyes . . . wriggling and turning like snakes. And see, what was that? One of the snakes seized its own tail and the image whirled scornfully before my eyes. As though from a flash of lightning I awoke. I occupied the rest of the night in working out the consequence of the hypothesis.

Kekulé had dreamed the ring (or closed-chain) theory of the benzene molecule, which made a major breakthrough in the chemistry of his day.

Examples of dream creation are numerous. Elias Howe received the idea for his eye-pointed sewing machine needle in his sleep. While dreaming that he was being threatened by savages, he noticed that the spears they were carrying had holes near the spear points — the solution he needed for the proper threading of a sewing machine needle. The composer Tartini heard the devil play a beautiful sonata in a dream and awoke to write down "The Devil's Trill" as he had heard it in his sleep. Richard Wagner credited a dream for the prelude to his opera, *Das Rheingold*, while Robert Louis Stevenson dreamed entire stories, including *The Strange Case of Dr. Jekyll and Mr. Hyde.*

Nor is dream invention reserved for men of the arts and sciences. Recently, a personal friend was unable to repair the cruise control in his car until he saw, in a dream, just how to do it. Another acquaintance said that since grade school he had developed the habit of working on problems in his sleep. His technique was to repeat the problem out loud three times just before turning in. Then he would forget about it, confident that his sleeping mind would work on the problem. In the morning, often while doing something else, he would find the solution "popping" into his mind.

## *New and Productive Patterns*

But does anything we have learned so far help us to discover the source of creative ideas? In one way, perhaps. An additional clue to the puzzle of inventiveness is emerging. While some imaginative people attempt to increase their inventive abilities by living unconventional lives or by getting help in dreams, each person has gotten novel ideas in his or her own field of expertise — poets receive inspiration in poetry, scientists find solutions to scientific problems, mechanics have flashes of insight on car repair. The fact that poets seem never to have visions about how to fix their carburetors leads modern theorists to speculate that creativity is *not* some random revelation given to us by supernatural forces, but only the mental shuffling of what we already know into new and productive patterns.

Certain kinds of modern sculpture can be used to provide a clear example of this "old into new" transformation. For instance, an artist-friend used to drive her Volkswagon to the salvage yard to pick up odd scraps of metal from which she fashioned her sculpture. The men at the yard (imagine what they thought about the artist) would weigh her car on the way in, then weigh the loaded car again on its exit in order to charge her for the additional pounds of scrap she was carrying off. In her workshop, of course, she was welding those bits and pieces of rusty iron into exotic sculptures of turtles, weight lifters, locomotives, and spaceships (one "Star Trek" creation featured a rusty spade blade as the hull of the ship). In this case, a creative mind recycled "junk" into sculpture.

Not until the new discipline of psychology began to study human behavior in a scientific way, however, was real progress made toward understanding the creative process of the human brain. Even then, gains came fitfully, as indicated by the research of the late nineteenth-century figure, Cesare Lombroso. In addition to his (long since discredited) ideas that criminals have certain physical characteristics by which they can be recognized — small, pointed ears; low foreheads; and close-set eyes — Lombroso felt that creative men have facial and bodily traits in common. He asserted that inventive people have a disproportionate number of the following physical weaknesses: a tendency toward such diseases as rickets, pale complexion, small and emaciated bodies, cretinlike faces, a tendency to stutter, left-handness, and sterility. Although certain creative men have had handicaps (Lord Byron was born with a clubfoot; Alexander Pope, the poet, and Toulouse-Lautrec, the painter, were dwarfish), the fact that some less than physi-

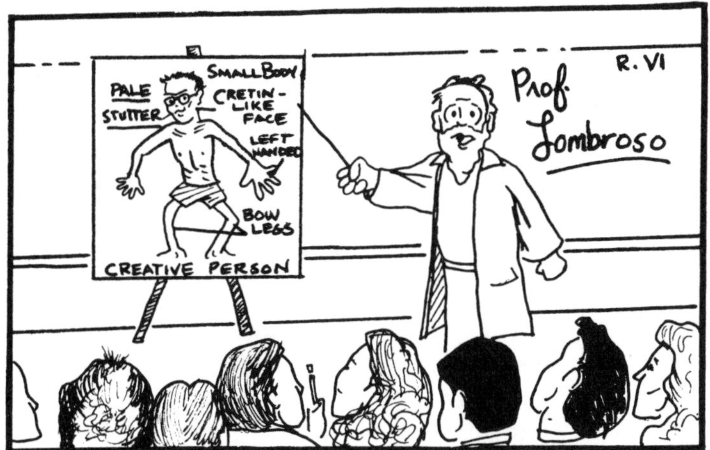

cally perfect humans make a living in the creative arts tells us nothing about what *produces* originality.

## Twentieth-Century Studies

The early twentieth-century reformer, Graham Wallas, got somewhat nearer the source of the creative process, which he outlines in his book, *The Art of Thought.* Summarizing his own and other people's work in this area, Wallas described four stages of creation.

The first stage he called *Preparation.* That is, the person expecting to gain new insights must know his field of study, be well prepared. This seems to fit what we have already seen; people get inventive ideas only in their own fields — poets, in poetry; scientists, in science.

Wallas called the second stage in the creative process *Incubation.* He noted that many great ideas came only after a period of time spent away from the problem. (This was certainly the experience of Archimedes.)

Wallas quoted Helmholtz, a leading physicist in the late nineteenth century, as saying, after he had investigated a problem, "in all directions... happy ideas come unexpectedly without effort, like an inspiration. So far as I was concerned, they have never come to me when my mind was fatigued, or when I was at my working table." Helmholtz is describing the experience common to many of getting an idea while doing something far removed from a problem — when walking or when mowing the lawn, for instance. This "click" or "flash" of a new idea is Wallas's third period of creativity, the *Illumination* stage. Click, flash, illumination? We're suddenly back to the same mysterious "dawning" of the new idea that puzzled the Greeks. Resting the mind by doing other activities was the only suggestion Wallas could offer about how creative ideas form.

The fourth and final step Wallas called *Verification,* making the necessary efforts to see if the "happy idea" actually solves the problem. Since "great" ideas don't always work out in actual practice, this final step is vitally important to the success of any original project.

More recently, Frank Barron made an attempt to get closer to the inventive process by studying people known for their creativity, primarily writers. In his book *Creative Person and Creative Process* (1969), he writes:

> Creation has long been thought of as a mystery and has been deemed the province of religion or, more broadly, of the supernatural.... This sense of the mystery surrounding creation is close to a universal sentiment, and certainly it may be found in the breasts of even the most scientific of psychologists as they approach the phenomenon of psychic creativity.

Unfortunately, in this passage we are again plunged back to mystery, almost to the gods, as the source of invention. Continuing, Barron says that creative writers speak "of the unconscious as the source of their important ideas and insights." Barron also notes that dreams seem to play a part in the imaginative process. The men and women he studied have "a more vivid dream life, with a notably greater tendency to have dreams in color, and also to have more nightmares; more hunches of an almost precognitive sort, and greater readiness to believe in prophetic dreams." He finds that persons of inventive genius tend to be "strange," but superior.

> From these data one might be led to conclude that creative writers are, as the common man has long suspected them to be, a bit "dotty." And of course it has always been a matter of pride in self-consciously artistic and intellectual circles to be, at the least, eccentric. "Mad as a hatter" is a term of high praise when applied to a person of marked intellectual endowments. But the "divine madness" that the Greeks considered a gift of the gods and an essential ingredient in the poet was not, like psychosis, something subtracted from normality; rather, it was something added. Genuine psychosis is stifling and imprisoning; the divine madness is a liberating from "the consenses."

So, where are we? Interpreting creativity as the product of the eccentric mind or praising it as the mark of the gifted does little to further our knowledge of it. And yet we have gained some understandings. We know that invention normally comes only in a person's field of specialization. Wallas is right when he says there must first be a Preparation stage; people have to become knowledgeable in some field before they may expect ideas to "dawn" on them in that area. (Probably the more we know, the more apt we are to get new ideas; novel ideas seem to come from a fortunate scrambling of information we already have.) And yet, although a certain threshold level of knowledge seems necessary for creativity, creative breakthroughs are not always the product of the most expert thinkers in a discipline (more on this later).

Ideas also seem to come after a period of Incubation—that is, rest, time spent away from the problem at hand. This Incubation period may be days, months, even years—or only a brief moment. When working on a math problem, for instance, a person is often stumped for a second or two before having an idea about a new and productive way to attack it. This new thought about how to proceed is as much an act of creation as an idea that "clicks" into place months later. So much less spectacular are "immediate ideas," flowing past from moment to moment, however, that they often go unrecognized for what they are—creative.

Two recent examples illustrate the effects of the Incubation period. Rob Fulop, a designer of electronic games, who spends time "kicking back and creating" at Lake Tahoe or Palm Springs, says his best ideas come to him when he is away from the office. This kind of "away from the office" inspirational idea occurred to an English engineer, R. Charles Draper, who came up with the concept for the design of the Thames Barrier Dam while cleaning Christmas decorations out of his garage. While doing that, he chanced to see a gas cock. The valve design caused him to imagine a movable floodgate shaped like a slice of the gas cock, flat on one side, rounded on the other; the idea was so simple and effective that it was immediately adopted.

Leaving aside Wallas's troubling third stage for the moment, let us examine the fourth step—Verification, or checking to see if the creative ideas actually work. Before Draper came up with the design for the Thames Barrier Dam, for instance, other creative suggestions that had been made were to blast in "a load of muddy goop to stop up the river temporarily," freeze part of the river like a skating rink, or build huge, ugly drop gates, "long flat slabs that would hang in the air suspended from three-hundred-foot towers." Each of these suggestions was creative enough, just not very practical, and certainly not as efficient as Draper's gas-cock idea. Muddy goop, skating rinks, and three-hundred-foot towers all failed the Verification stage of Wallas's four-part description of the creative process.

Returning to Wallas's third step, Inspiration, we find that *it* is the sticking point—as it has been throughout history. Neither Wallas nor anyone else has been able to explain just how to *control* inspiration. Even the most creative have found inspiration a fragile and elusive quality. Consider the case of the philosopher Immanuel Kant. Staring out his window one day, Kant realized he was unable to concentrate because a tree had grown up in his line of sight, changing the view he was accustomed to. Blocked by this slight change in his ritualistic (sight-thought) pattern, Kant could think of nothing to free his mind but to ask his neighbor to chop down the offending tree!

And so we find that people have waited for the gods to provide creativity or led unconventional lives as a way of "freeing up the mind." Artists, dancers, actors, and poets have lived in cold-water, walk-up apartments, moved to the Left Bank in Paris, or adopted unusual life styles (Bohemian, Beatnik, or Hippy, for instance)—all as a way of courting flashes of creative insight. And some truly creative individuals have led rather peculiar lives—Shelley, Byron, Galton. Still, the fact remains that adopting "strange life styles" does not seem to generate creativity for the vast majority of people.

Drugging out the rational mind has even been tried; people use alcohol, opium, marijuana, LSD (and every other stimulant and depressant imaginable). But even if people wish to risk their reputation by adopting "wild" life styles or their health by taking drugs, it has yet to be proved that these methods increase creativity. People on drugs sometimes do say these chemicals enhance their inventive powers, but then the last person apt to be rational enough to *know* is someone on drugs. Most drunks are convinced they are clever, handsome, and charming, though their sober friends know better.

The truth is that, from the Greeks to today, no one has been able to provide a system that will help men and women have inventive ideas at will. Desperate to find the mental source of creativity, a westerner might turn to oriental philosophy only to scurry back to western science upon hearing of years and years of silent meditation as a necessary first step to enlightenment. No one has that kind of time; this is America, the land of the free and the home of McDonald's; this is the place where everyone agrees the first thing to do with a balky piece of machinery is give it a swift kick. Surely there is a way, without fooling with drugs, to give the creative part of the human mind that swift kick, shoulder it forward, get it in gear. Perhaps if we just knew more about the brain...

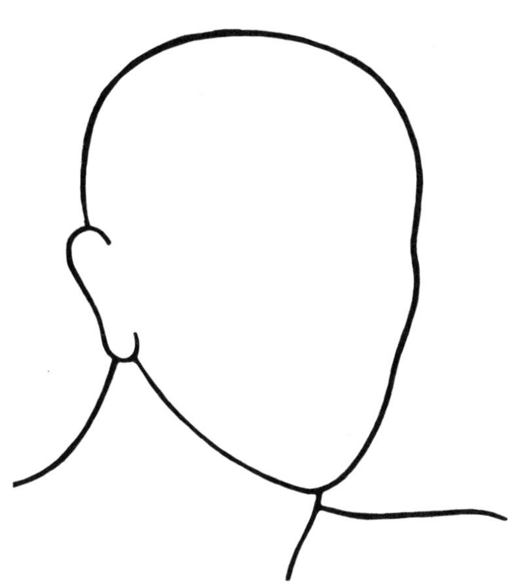

# 2
# About the Brain

*"I feel like I'm coming apart at the seams."*
*"I've got to get my head together."*
*"I'm of two minds about that."*

When you use one of these clichés, do you want people to think you actually have *two* minds? Of course not. No matter how much we might feel "all in pieces," each of us believes he or she is a "whole" person, with a unique personality. The words I, me, and mine litter our conversation. We are *ourselves* and, if asked, can describe *us* in great detail. We know what we like — Beethoven, tutti-frutti ice cream, hardwood floors, French kissing — and what we don't like — roaches, grits, sweaty palms, and rings around our collars. Each of us is a walking clutter of economic, political, religious, and social ideas by which we describe ourselves *to* ourselves and to others. We have undergone changes, of course, no longer enjoy certain foods or colors as we once did, fallen in and out of love, even switched political parties or religions. Still, each of us believes he has a fixed core of personality that, four years of age or forty, has never changed. We may be indecisive at times, but we believe our head *is* together, that we *are* of one mind. Right? . . . Well, *maybe*!

"Things are not always what they seem."

"All things are possible."

"There are more things in heaven and earth, Horatio, than are dreamt of in your philosophy."

Reminded by these old adages that nothing is as illusory as certainty, we will now consider what modern science has discovered about the human brain.

It has been known for some time that man's higher brain (neocortex) is divided into two, roughly similar segments called the left brain (on the left-hand side of the body) and the right brain (on the other side). By examining accident victims and stroke patients, doctors have noticed curiosities in the operation of the left and right brain. Contrary to what might seem likely, we now know that, basically, the right half of the brain controls the left side of the body; the left half, the right side.

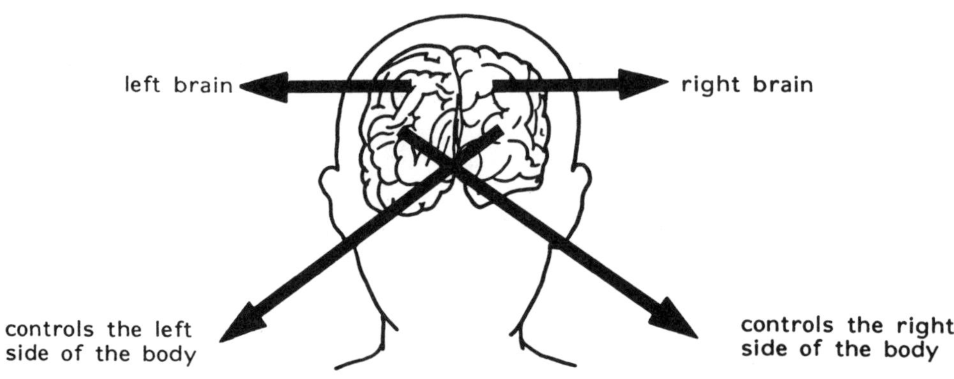


back view

As early as 1836, a French doctor reported another surprising finding: impairment of his patients' left brains caused them to lose their ability to speak, while similar harm to their right brains did not. In the 1940s, additional discoveries about brain function led doctors to consider surgery as a way to stop seizures in Grand Mal epileptics. Physicians reasoned that the irregular brain activity that produced convulsions would be interrupted if the connective tissue between the left and right brains was severed. Cutting the links between left and right brains of humans did reduce seizures, and the epileptic patients recovered to function normally. Well, not *quite* normally. Strange behavior sometimes occurred, indicating that not only the patients' brains but also their bodies had been fractured into left and right. When getting ready to go to work, for instance, one "split-brain" patient found one of his hands busily buttoning up his shirt while the other (driven by the opposite side of the brain) was just as eagerly unbuttoning the shirt. Without his being aware of it, one hand was acting as if it "wished" to go to work, the other as though it "wanted" to stay home. Because the two brain halves could no longer communicate with each other, one hand (or more correctly "brain") literally did not know what the other was doing! In yet another instance, a patient reached out to grab a pretty woman while his other hand seized the offending hand, to stop such uncivilized behavior.

Intrigued by these findings, scientists began devising ways to test split-brain patients in an attempt to learn more about how surgery affected these patients. Allowed to see a picture with only the left-brain visual field, a split-brain patient could tell the researcher, "This is a picture of a cow." But if the patient saw the same picture with only the right-brain visual field, he could not speak about it at all. The split-brain patient could form no words even though he could point to a similar picture of a cow, showing that he had recognized the image. (The passage of time moderated some of the more bizarre reactions of split-brain people. You will be pleased to learn that such surgery is rarely performed today, however; drugs have been proved a more effective treatment.)

Research continues on accident victims, though, and on patients who must have one-half of the brain anesthetized in preparation for surgery. These studies have increased our knowledge about the specialized functions of the left and right brains. The left side of the brain has a marked tendency to control logical thinking and is responsible for the step-by-step development of the thought process. For the most part, the left side also controls language and is the symbolic side of the brain. Furthermore, it is generally the dominant side, suppressing the right brain so completely that it often seems to be our complete "self."

The functions of the right side of the brain present quite a different picture. Compared to the left side, the right seems undisciplined, mystical, pictorial, and "creative." In particular, the right side is able to unite seemingly unrelated bits of information into an integrated pattern, much as a mosaic design is produced by arranging colored bits of stone into a picture. In this ability, the right brain is the *pattern seeker,* constantly shifting and sorting the data of experience into a variety of patterns that it offers to the left side of the brain as a means for making sense out of the world. Whereas the right brain is the *pattern seeker,* the left brain serves as the *pattern user.* From the multitude of patterns suggested by the right brain, the left brain uses its function of logical thought to select the one it thinks will work best in a given situation. And so we can see that a beneficial relationship characterizes left-right brain interactions. The right brain suggests various ways of interpreting the world, and the left brain picks the pattern it feels is best. The following diagram shows what has been suggested so far about the tendencies of the brain's two sides.

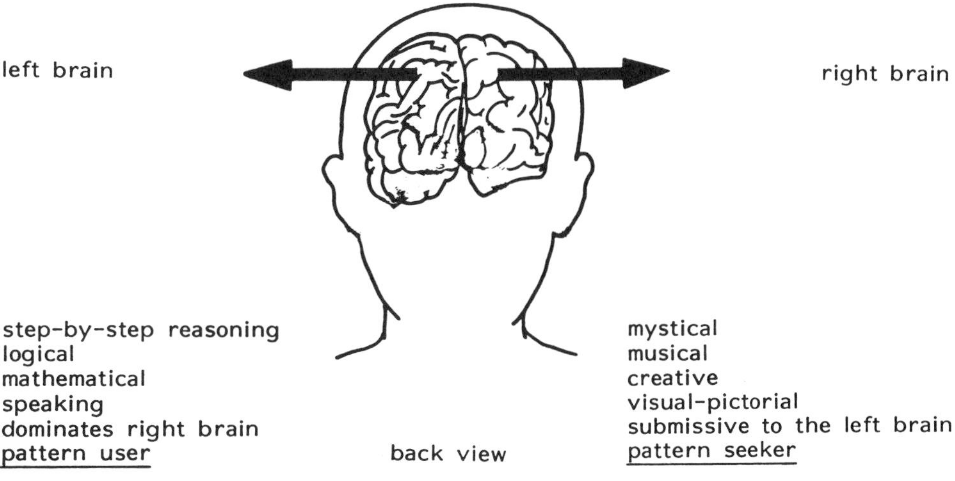

## The Power of Patterns

Most of the time, we rely on our "reasonable" left brain to find logical solutions to our problems and to keep us out of danger. Speculation is that the left brain (either by direct experience or from having absorbed the wisdom of others) memorizes patterns of what it considers to be good or bad. The left brain then matches any new information it receives to these "experience patterns" to help us make decisions in new situations. In this way, we (and other animals) are pattern-following creatures. Those organisms "fittest to survive" are the ones recognizing patterns well enough that once clawed by a "tiger" they can recognize similarities between *all* "tigers" and avoid the entire species.

The left brain has learned a number of "truths" (established patterns) and is simply not happy unless it can match new information to these old certainties. (For instance, when you see an unfamiliar metal object in your driveway, isn't your mind uneasy until you have fitted that... thing... into some known pattern? Don't you begin searching your memory banks by saying to yourself, "I wonder if that dropped off my car? It doesn't look valuable. Maybe it's from a sewing machine?" In the same vein, a loud sound will drive all other thoughts from our mind until we have identified it — fit it into a pattern.) This patterning behavior is good for us most of the time. We don't have to experiment with each new "tiger" before running away from it or, more relevant to the modern world, knowing the effect of alcohol, we refuse to ride with a drunk driver.

Unfortunately, our affection for patterns often makes it difficult for us to reject an established pattern and accept new ideas. But if the left brain were not rigid about its concept of truth, we might be subject to disturbing flip-flops in our view of the world. It would be dangerous, for instance, to be driving a car and suddenly decide that the car was stationary and the road was moving. The prospect of having no control over the speed of the *road* would be terrifying! Even the evidence of our senses must occasionally be modified by the previous patterns the left brain has learned. (No matter how it looks, experience tells us that distant water on a dry road is a mirage.) No doubt a prehistoric man in an elevator, not understanding the pattern of elevators, would be easily confused by his experience. Only able to feel the elevator's speed through its brief period of acceleration, he would probably conclude he had been transported to the eighteenth floor by magic!

In review, we now think the left side of the brain is responsible for step-by-step reasoning, logic, mathematical ability, and speaking; it is the part of the brain that defends the patterns by which a person makes sense out of the world. (It will hurt to fall off that cliff; you might be in an accident, so wear clean underwear.) In effect, the left brain gives the world a consistent organization.

By contrast, the right side of the brain is the "wild" side of the intellect — mystical, pictorial, and creative. Whereas the left brain defends the patterns it recognizes, the right side forms new patterns from stray bits of information. As the submissive part of the brain, however, the right side is often prevented from "doing its own thing" by the logical, but somewhat "prim," left brain. The right brain constantly suggests new patterns of the world; the left brain seldom deigns to

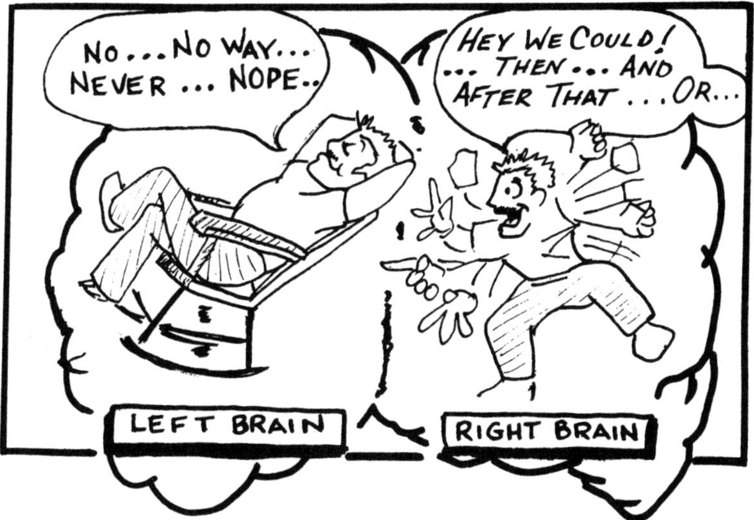


consider any of them. Returning to the theme of this book — creativity — we now see that the right brain plays a crucial role in *making new patterns*. And making new patterns in the mind is, after all, what we call *creativity*!

With the logical left brain defending old, sensible patterns by refusing even to recognize new designs generated by the right brain, it's no wonder inventive ideas dawn on us so rarely. To continue with our "driving" example, we can see why it's all well and good for the left brain to refuse to admit the possibility that the car is stationary on a moving road, but this idea may be *precisely* what an electronics wizard needs to produce a road-race game. Arcade racing games feature the driver's car in a fixed position on the playing screen. The car can move only laterally on the game's electronic road; the road moves *under* the car. In short, to be creative, we must be able to imagine the "unthinkable."

It seems that the brain is both "naturally creative" and "naturally non-creative"! Our right brain's constant generation of a wide assortment of patterns is obviously a creative enterprise, but the left brain's natural tendency to select and use one pattern blocks this spontaneous creativity. The left brain's defensiveness is normally beneficial since it gives us a consistent view of the world. When we need to be creative, however, this defensiveness serves instead to frustrate our efforts.

Still, the right brain does occasionally penetrate the left brain's "status quo" defenses. How? At times, the left brain's passion for consistent organization eases up when its old patterns don't seem to be working in actual practice, much as someone in the desert not finding water in its usual forms will begin having ideas about eating moist plants, a possibility that would never be considered under other circumstances. Though rare, getting a wonderfully illuminating idea that explains events or untangles a snarl better than any previously attempted approaches is an experience most of us have had. (Some call this an "aha" experience.) Suddenly a fresh pattern (which we believe the right brain provides) comes to mind.

We "believe" the right brain is linked to creative ideas, but can we prove this? The best evidence, of course, would be if, somehow, we could all "feel" the right brain getting an idea. But this simply doesn't happen, so even the "naturally creative" person finds it difficult to explain *exactly* how a creative idea forms. This may be because the left brain, with its step-by-step thinking, can recognize the arrival of a new idea, but not comprehend its source ("It just popped into my head!"). Conversely, the right brain, while possessing the ability to create new patterns, lacks the verbal talent and dominance to make the individual "aware" of the particulars of the creative process. As a result, the act of creation, even for those skilled at it, retains a mysterious and *unconscious* aura.

## But Is the Mystery Unsolvable?

We think not. While there may be no direct, personal verification of the right brain's role in creativity, the premise that the right brain is linked to inventiveness is supported by far more than mere speculation. When comparing the earlier discussion of historical attempts to understand inventiveness to our current knowledge of the brain, for instance, we see some interesting connections.

| *Historical View* | *Present Knowledge of the Right Brain* |
|---|---|
| Mystic states lead to creativity. | Right brain associated with mystic states. |
| Ideas come "out of the blue." | Right brain linked to the unconscious. |
| Ideas come in dreams. | Right brain connected to dreaming. |
| Creativity linked to abnormal states. | Normal left-brain dominance must be overcome to allow right-brain input. |
| Inventive solutions flash as pictures. | Right brain is pictorial. |
| Creative people are unconventional. | Right brain opposite of conventional left brain. |

We can now see how well earlier ideas about the *source* of creativity fit into our present understanding of the *right brain*. While the ancient Greeks attributed their inspiration to *mystical* visits of the *gods*, creative breakthroughs probably originated much closer to home — in the right brain, which (coincidentally?) has been linked to mystical states and *unconscious* perceptions. When earlier poets felt, intuitively, that conventional society stifled their inventive impulses, it was really the left (conventional) side of the brain that was blocking off novel ideas from consciousness. Why is the left brain linked with societal conventions? The conventions or "rules" of society are simply those *patterns* that most people find desirable most of the time (wearing clothing, eating with silverware, shaking hands when meeting, etc.).

And what of some people getting ideas in their sleep, in their dreams? Could this be because sleep seems to affect the left side of the mind more than the right side? (Sleep investigators have found that the "sleeping" right brain is more active than the "sleeping" left brain.) Speculation is that the right brain has dreams that seep into the left brain when the left is too drowsy to dominate the right brain as it normally would. Coleridge's dreams of "pleasure domes" and "sacred rivers," Kekulé's "benzene snake," and Tartini's "Devil's Trill" may well be right-brain patterns that drifted into the "sleeping" left brain.

Considering this information, it is tempting to assume that the right brain is *synonymous* with creativity. But this would be an exaggeration. It is probably better to say that the right brain is responsible for the most significant part of the creative endeavor (Wallas's Illumination stage), using its *pattern-seeking* abilities to shuffle old information into new configurations. Of equal importance, though, are Wallas's stages of Preparation and Verification, states in which the individual, using the left brain, first gains knowledge, then applies creative "solutions" to the world to verify their worth. In Verification, for instance, many truly creative ideas—such as freezing the Thames or blocking it with muddy goop—will be found to be stupid, impractical, or off-the-wall and will be discarded as unworkable. If you ignore the logical left brain, you may find yourself acting on some "fun" suggestion from the right brain about jumping off a ten-story building with umbrella in hand, not a pleasant prospect. It follows that nothing of practical value is apt to happen unless your reasoning mind can sort through the right brain's imaginings.

Combining what we now know about brain function with Wallas's four stages of creativity, we can see how *both* sides of the brain are involved in the inventive process:

| | |
|---|---|
| *Preparation:* | left brain acquires knowledge. |
| *Incubation:* | right brain works on patterns; left brain relaxes. |
| *Illumination:* | right brain translates answer to left brain. |
| *Verification:* | left brain tries out the possible solution and evaluates it. |

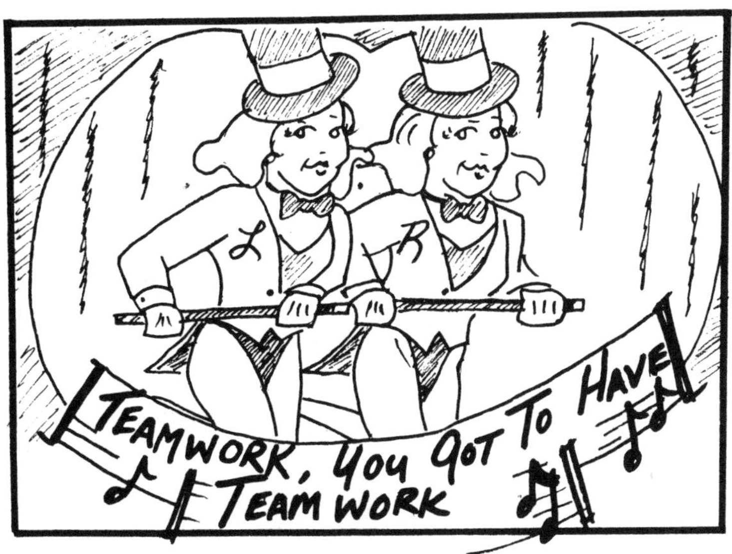

## *Not a Mystery but a Barrier*

Our insights into the brain suggest that creativity is not the province of the few but a condition that *everyone* has the potential to develop. We could even say that inventiveness could become a normal mental process of left- and right-brain interaction. If this hypothesis is correct, the solution to our creativity problems seems easy. We simply need to have the proper relationship between the two sides of the brain for creativity to result. So why don't we all develop that relationship? . . . Because it's hard! It is difficult to be inventive because real, tangible barriers block creativity. For one thing, as already mentioned, the left brain tends to ignore input from the right. (This genetic dominance is not complete, however, and would probably not of itself block inventiveness.) A more difficult bar, perhaps, is a *social* one. Simply stated, though society *seems* to applaud the creative person, in reality it expends considerable effort *blocking* creativity. Society is devoted to stressing left-brain skills in schools, to encouraging the memorization of the *right answer*, or THE TRUTH. How many courses stress the importance of finding *new* approaches to problems rather than just memorizing old solutions? Hardly any. Most education is based on society's collective left brain perpetuating the old patterns society values. Some old answers work well, of course. It is just that a consistent emphasis on THE TRUTH prevents people from developing mental flexibility. As a result, new and creative patterns are seldom discovered by people who somehow have been made to feel it is WRONG to search for new ways to solve a problem.

Do you remember an earlier statement that creative breakthroughs are often achieved by those who, though knowledgeable, are not the top scholars in a field? Can you guess why? It may be because those who have learned *the most* about a particular discipline have been so successful in knowing THE TRUTH that to veer away from this established pattern of knowledge would be a threat to their image, their prestige. Often those less ingrained, therefore, those less rigid in their certainty of THE TRUTH are the ones who find *new* molds into which TRUTH is again recast.

And what is the fate of those few individuals who risk society's "slings and arrows" while undertaking new approaches to problem-solving? If society pays attention to them at all, they are labeled crackpots or, at best, dreamers . . . until . . . someone *else* discovers that the creator's ideas actually work. Only then is the artist (inventor, scientist) rewarded. After coming late to the recognition of a person's original contributions, society tends to overreact, and the GREAT individual is hailed as some sort of superhuman genius, a completely different person from you and me, a person who has that special "gift" of inventive genius.

For an example of how ideas about the creative person can become distorted, we have only to take a quick look at the career of Edward Jenner (1749 – 1823), England's creator of the smallpox vaccine. Making a successful inoculation in 1796, Jenner did not receive wide recognition in his own country until he had gained a considerable reputation on the continent. Years later, having overcome his critics at home, he was recognized by Parliament, which gave him a £10,000 grant. Although it may seem odd that Jenner was not given early support

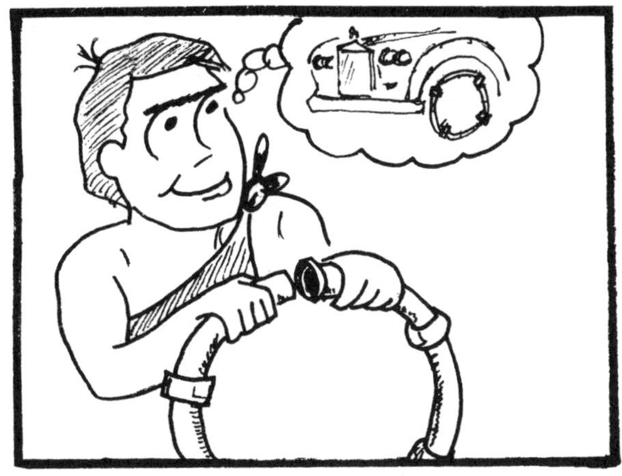

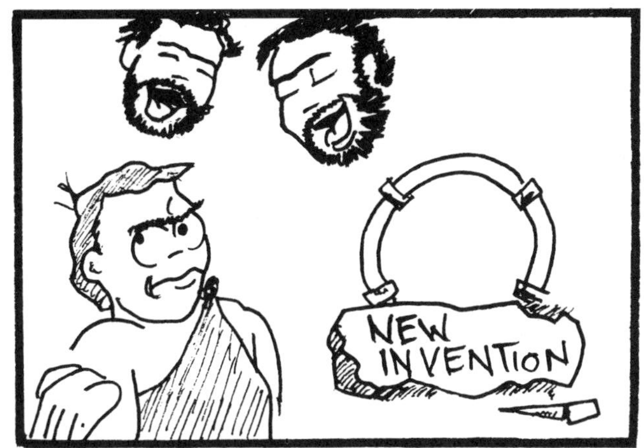
NEW
INVENTION

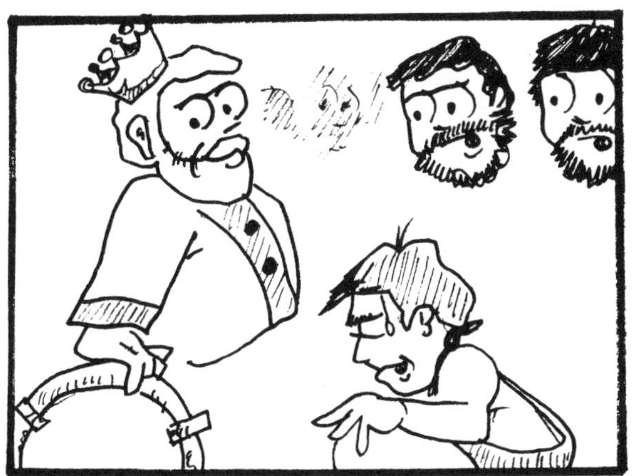

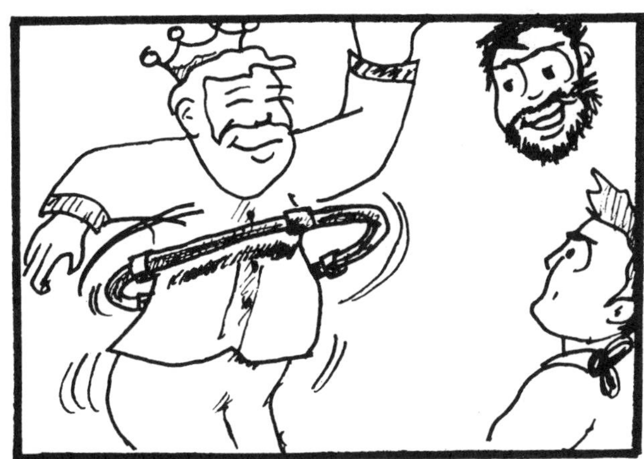

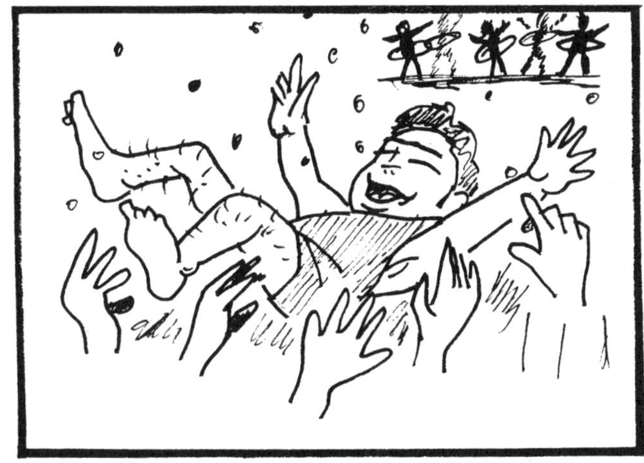

at home, even stranger is Jenner's current reputation as a medical genius, stemming as it does from an observation that was common knowledge to England's milkmaids: people previously infected with cowpox did not contract smallpox.

In view of Jenner's situation, notice how the system works to discourage creativity. First, society tells people they are wrong to look for creative approaches, either ridiculing or ignoring those who try and seem to fail. Then, if by some good fortune a person is recognized as successful, that person is elevated to such a lofty status that the rest of us think it is useless to try to become such GREAT THINKERS! And in these attitudes is the implied message that creativity is a special gift that can't be taught, can't be developed. We disagree! *Our* investigations show that creativity is not "magic," but the result of increased interplay between the right and left brain. While a few — the "naturally creative" — have somehow developed this brain interaction on their own, our research indicates that the rest of us can also become inventive by using LARC, the *L*eft *A*nd *R*ight *C*reativity system we teach you, step-by-step, in Part II.

# part II
# Learning LARC

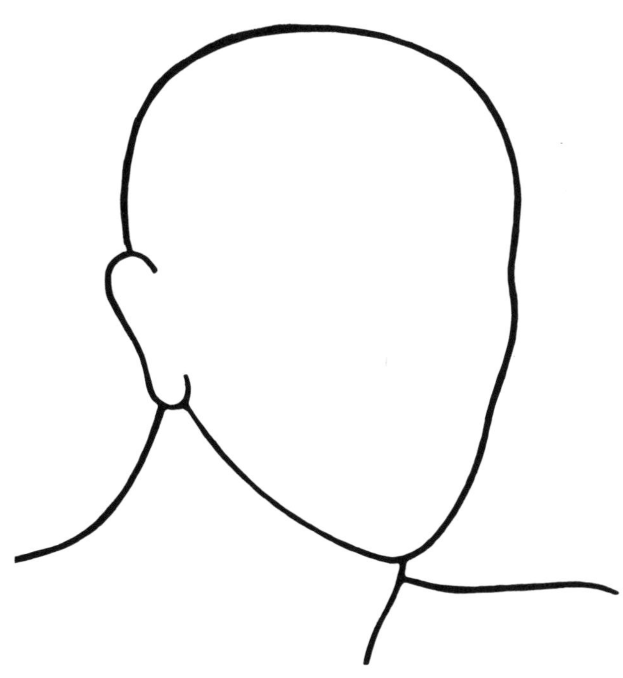

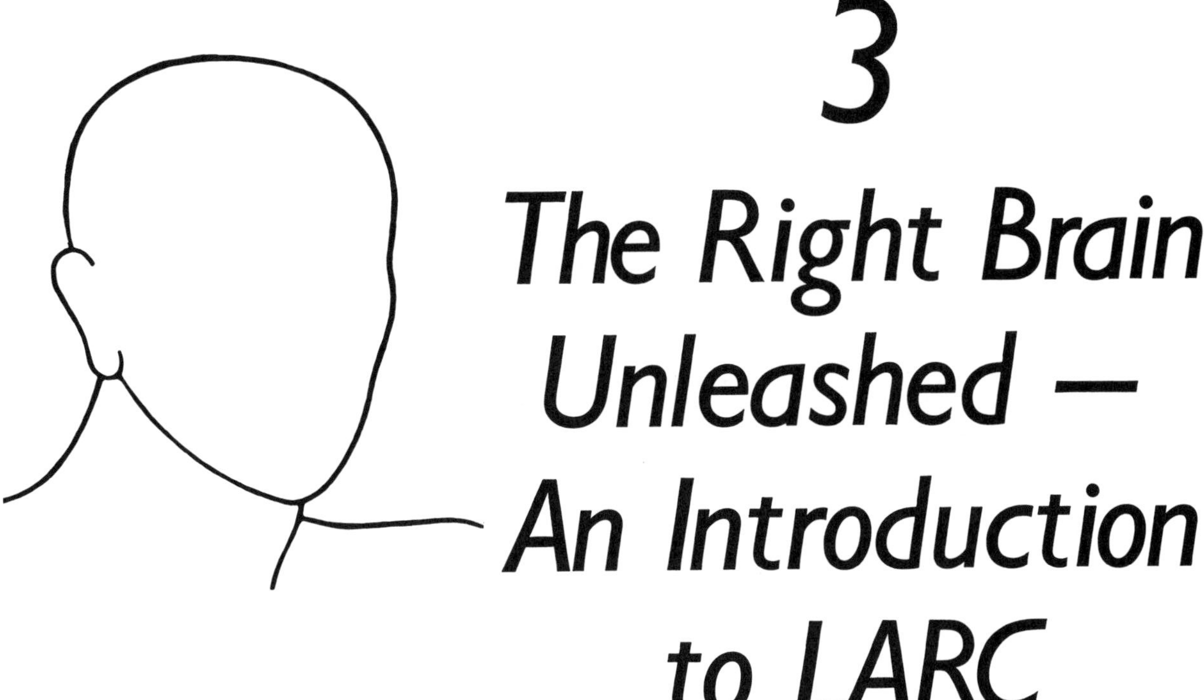

# 3 The Right Brain Unleashed — An Introduction to LARC

Before introducing LARC, let us address an important question. Is it really possible to make the "hard of hearing" left brain listen to the inventive suggestions of the "soft spoken" right brain? Yes. In fact, it has been done before in several *specific* areas.

## Creativity and Art

In her book, *Drawing on the Right Side of the Brain,* Betty Edwards suggests techniques for keeping the logical, verbal left brain from blocking off the creative visions of the pictorial right brain. While teaching drawing, Ms. Edwards kept having the following experience:

> I have always done a lot of demonstration drawing in my classes, and it was my wish during the demonstrations to explain to students what I was doing — what I was looking at, why I was drawing things in certain ways. I often find, however, that I would simply stop talking right in the middle of a sentence. I would hear my voice stop and I would think of getting back to the sentence, but finding the words again would seem like a terrible chore — and I didn't really want to anyway.

Her experience, a common one with artists, is that the "words" of her left brain get in the way of the nonverbal, but creative, right brain. She advises art students:

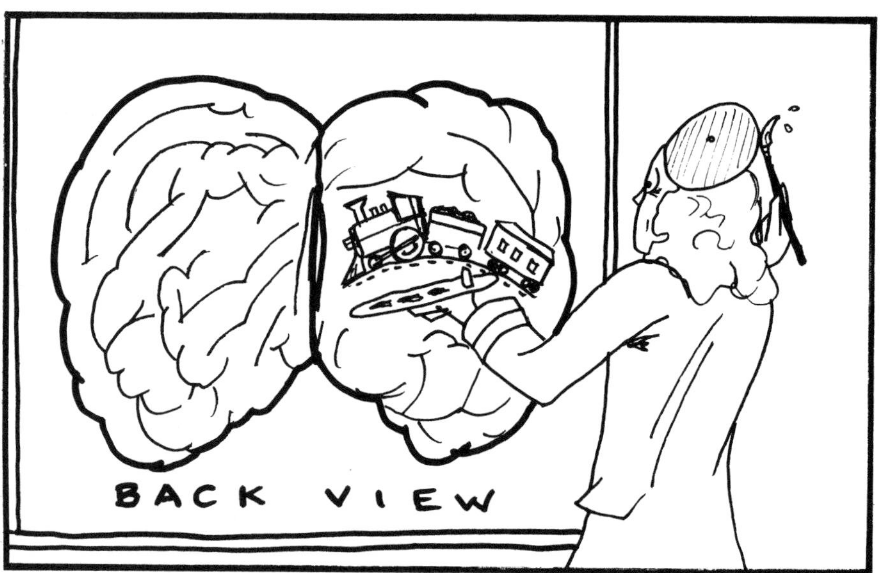


*Drawing on the right side of the brain.*

> . . . to direct your attention toward visual information that the left brain cannot or will not process. In other words, you will always try to present your brain with a task the left brain will refuse, thus allowing your right brain to use its capability for drawing.

LARC also triggers the right brain, but in a more general way, by producing a constant switching between right and left brains. Edwards continues:

> This yearning to quiet the L-mode [Edwards' symbol for the left brain] may practically explain centuries-old practices such as meditation and self-induced altered states of consciousness achieved through fasting, drugs, chanting, and alcohol."

Sound familiar? It should, since a similar sentiment was expressed in chapter 1. As for "centuries-old practices such as meditation," how about the famous Zen meditation question: "You know the sound of two hands clapping. What is the sound of one hand clapping?" To the dominant left brain, of course, a problem like this is utter nonsense; the logical left brain refuses even to consider it. But the "wild and crazy" right brain would probably enjoy playing with such an enigma and coming up with who-knows-what inventive notions.

## Blind Man's Comb

Another way to trigger the right brain's input was discovered, quite by chance, by one of this book's authors. While walking through the neighborhood, he saw a tin can about fifteen feet ahead of him on the sidewalk. Just for fun, he decided to picture in his mind the can's location, then closed his eyes and walked forward to see if he could come close to stepping on the can. Rather surprisingly, he thought, he hit the can — the can's position was exactly where his mental picture said it should be. It then occurred to him that forming a visual image of the can's location was strongly "right brain" in nature.

Soon, using a comb instead of a can, he had others trying this simple experiment. Interestingly, different people had differing levels of success. Eyes closed, some walked swiftly to the comb, stepping on it with unerring accuracy. Others, even when measuring their steps carefully, going slowly, counting under their breaths, would miss the mark — often quite badly. Those failing to hit the target often talked of calculating the distance to the comb, of counting paces (such mathematical systems are the special province of the left brain). Though it made "sense" to do it that way, "counting systems" just didn't seem to work well at all. But when the counters switched to visualizing the comb's location in their "mind's eye," then closed their eyes and walked to where they "saw" it, their performances improved dramatically. So what was happening? Basically, solving the problem of stepping on the comb blindfolded is not accomplished by logical, "thinking" approaches but by imagining, in a picture, how far away that pesky comb lies. Like the work of Betty Edwards, this "step on the comb" illustration demonstrates that *some* problems are best solved by "unleashing the right brain's" responses.

## The Right Brain for the Inner Game

While the "comb" example demonstrating the right brain's knack for performing physical tasks is enlightening, a more important investigation of brain function as it relates to physical skills was undertaken by W. Timothy Gallwey in his books *The Inner Game of Tennis* and *Inner Tennis — Playing the Game.*

As a tennis instructor, Gallwey noticed several interesting things about his students. For one, he found that *showing* them how to play worked better than *telling* them what to do. (Betty Edwards teaches her art students in a similar manner.) For another, Gallwey noticed that the harder his pupils tried, the *worse they played.* A player who looked "loose" in practice would "tighten up" in a match, "choking" on the big points. This last observation is a common one, of course, familiar to anyone who has ever played sports or sung a solo in church or read a poem before the entire first grade. "Choking," especially for amateurs, is a very human thing to do.

As for professionals, Gallwey talked to several leading tennis stars after they played particularly well, asking them how they did it, what they felt during the match, what they thought about as they played. Their answers? They said they had just been "on" that day. They talked about "playing out of their minds" or making "unconscious" shots. (Even we amateurs have had the delightful experience, from time to time, of "playing over our heads.") When Gallwey asked specifically about their thoughts, they replied that they were just playing, not *thinking* about much of anything.

Gallwey decided that players who talked to themselves while playing—coaching themselves by saying, "Get the racket back," "Move to the ball," "Make a higher toss," or, in utter despair after flubbing an easy shot, "You dummy! You've got to concentrate!"—actually did worse than those who just played with little conscious thought and *no* intellectual chatter. To Gallwey it seemed each player had two personalities, which he labeled *Self 1* and *Self 2*. Gallwey equated Self 1 with the mind, which thinks it knows all about how to play the game and shouts orders all the time. Self 2 is the "body," which actually knows how to play but is thrown off by constant criticism from the mind. What? The lowly body can play better than the exalted mind? Doesn't the body do only what the mind tells it to? Not for complex physical things, Gallwey thinks, reminding us that children learn to walk by seeing and mimicking, long before their minds have learned to shout orders. Apparently, the "body" can do new and complex things without constant supervision by the "mind."

Deciding that the mind was actually interfering with the body's ability to play tennis, Gallwey devised his Bounce-Hit system. He told his students to say *bounce* whenever the ball bounced on the court and *hit* when either they or their opponents hit the ball. Bounce-hit, bounce-hit, bounce-hit. But what good did saying bounce-hit do? It gave Self 1 (a person's verbal mentality) something to do. The mind wanted to say something so Gallwey gave it something harmless to say, something that did not interfere with the "body" playing the game. The result?

> The player loses himself in the action, continually breaking the false limits placed on his potential. Awareness becomes acutely heightened, while analysis anxiety and self-conscious thought are completely forgotten. Enjoyment is at a peak—pure and unspoiled.

By this time, what Gallwey calls Self 1 and Self 2 should sound familiar to you, particularly if you substitute left brain and right brain. When you think about it, hitting a tennis ball is rather creative, every shot forcing the player to form a new pattern of movement to be successful. It's a form of ballet in its requirement for synchronized body movement as patterns shift moment by moment.

Visual, pictorial, pattern-making, every shot requiring some new variation? These sound like right brain activities, don't they? In fact, we can speculate that it is not the "body" that knows how to play, but the right brain. And Gallwey's Self 1, shouting orders, confident in knowing all the answers, refusing to let the right brain do its best? Of course. It's the old, dominant, noncreative, orthodox left brain.

In answer to the question, "Is it really possible to make the 'hard of hearing' left brain listen to the inventive suggestions of the 'soft spoken' right brain?" we offer Edwards and Gallwey's experiences as evidence that techniques can be devised to keep the left brain "out of the way" of the creative right brain. Though both Edwards and Gallwey have discovered ingenious ways to "outwit" the left brain in *specific* areas—art and tennis—LARC is designed to help people become more inventive in *any* problem-solving activity they undertake.

Enough of examples, background, and demonstrations! It's time to explain LARC.

## An Overview of LARC (Left And Right Creativity)

Convinced by now that the right brain can be stimulated, you have only to see how to do this, not for artistic or athletic purposes, but for creative thinking in general. You will learn how to become more creative through LARC, a series of exercises that stimulates the right brain and causes the sorts of right-left interactions that produce not only inventive, but also *workable,* ideas.

*LARC: four versions.* To maximize its value, we present LARC in four versions—LARC I through IV—each a complete system for the stimulation of creative ideas. LARC I and II are quick sets of exercises that can prompt imaginative solutions to many problems. LARC III and IV are more complex, take more time, and are to be used for more difficult problems or when it is necessary to find even more inventive ideas than those produced by LARC I and II.

*Help in deciding which version should be used.* An analogy may be helpful. If you think of LARC as a mechanic's toolbox, LARC I would contain the basic tools a person would need to make minor adjustments to a car. LARC II would have the same tools as are in the first box plus a few extra ones necessary for slightly more involved repairs. Finally, LARC toolboxes III and IV, while still having all the apparatus contained in the earlier boxes, would also have special gadgets needed for a complete overhaul, everything necessary to work on that special, but temperamental, sports car. So what kinds of tools do *you* need to "tune up" your creativity? Most of the time, those contained in the LARC I or LARC II boxes will do the job. But the extra tools of LARC III and IV are provided—just in case.

While there are no mandatory rules regarding which LARC variation you choose, we suggest that you begin working on a problem with LARC I or LARC II. If they produce the inventive idea you need—great! If not, then try again, using LARC III and IV.

*Learning LARC.* Learning LARC is relatively easy. After learning the simplest program—LARC I—you will be pleasantly surprised to discover that LARC II adds only a few more steps. This pattern continues; LARC III expands on LARC II, and LARC IV adds just a couple of new techniques.

*LARC summarized.* Outlined on the next page are the four LARC versions. Although the terminology will not be meaningful to you yet, you can see how each successive LARC uses the steps of earlier versions and adds only a few features of its own.

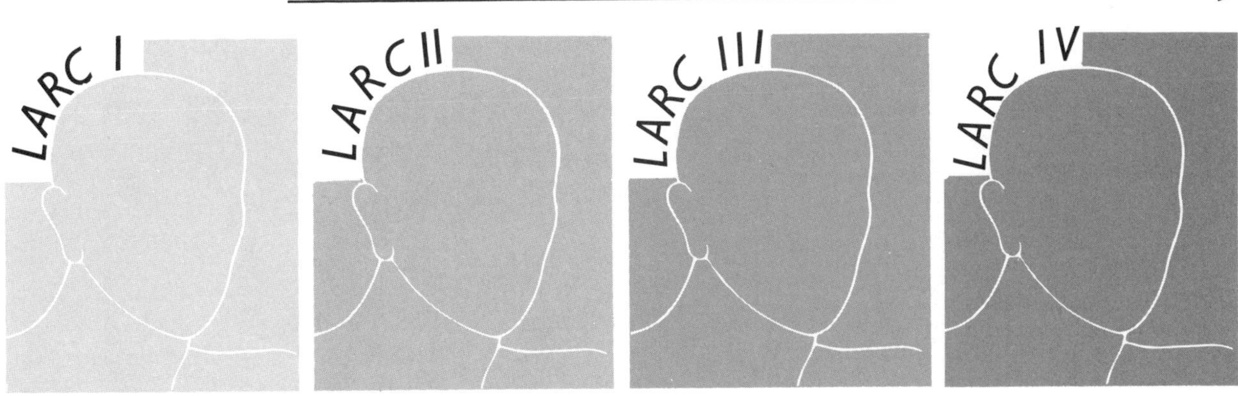

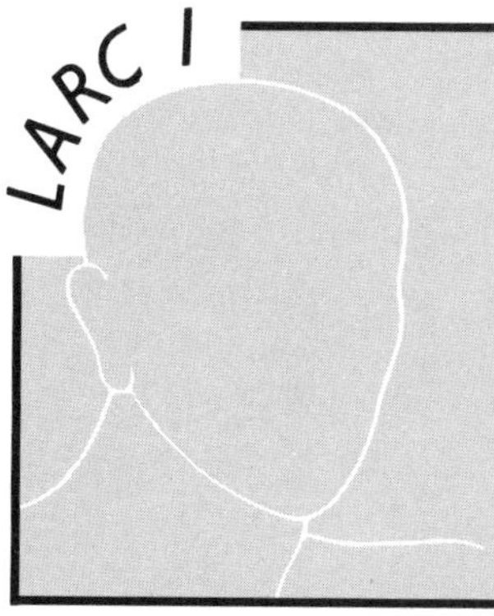

## LARC I

1. Drawing
2. Smashing
3. Creating I

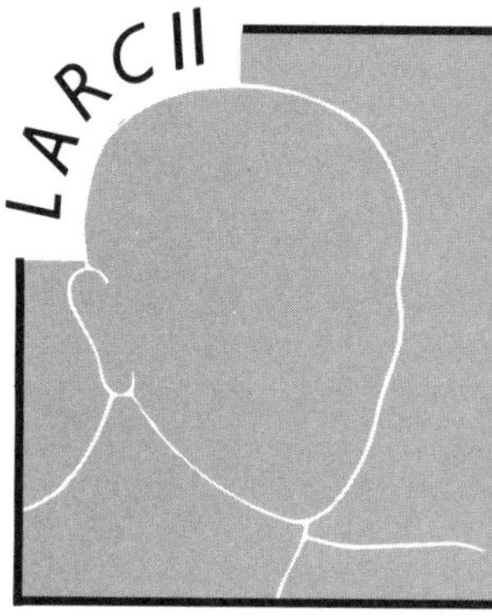

## LARC II

1. Drawing
2. Smashing
3. Creating I
4. Rearranging
5. Creating II

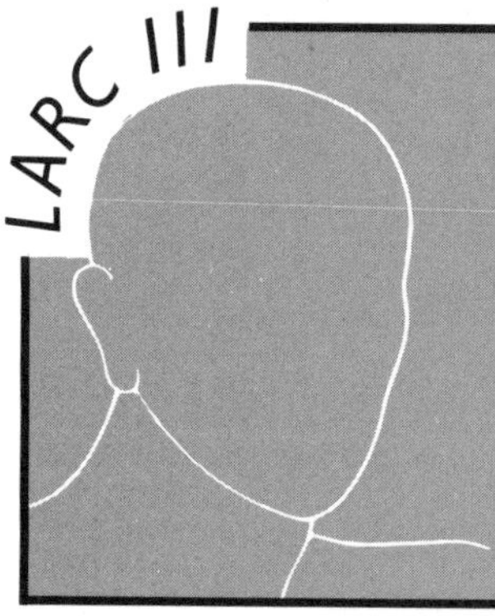

## LARC III

1. Drawing
2. Smashing
3. Creating I
4. Rearranging: Group, Pyramid, Chain, Circle
5. Creating II

## LARC IV

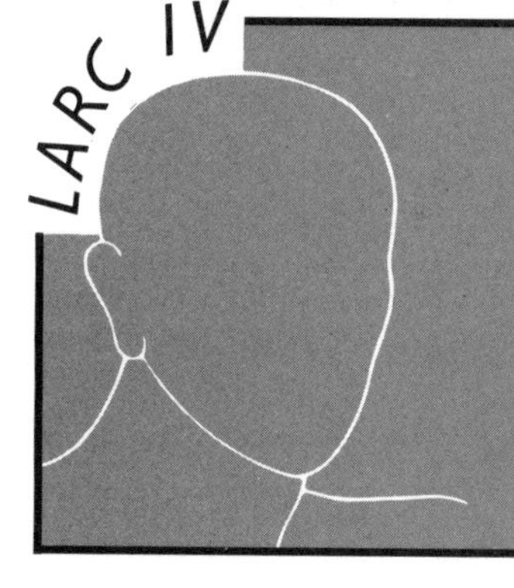

1. Stating the Problem
2. Drawing
3. Smashing
4. Creating I
5. Rearranging: Group, Pyramid, Chain, Circle
6. Creating II: Relationship lines

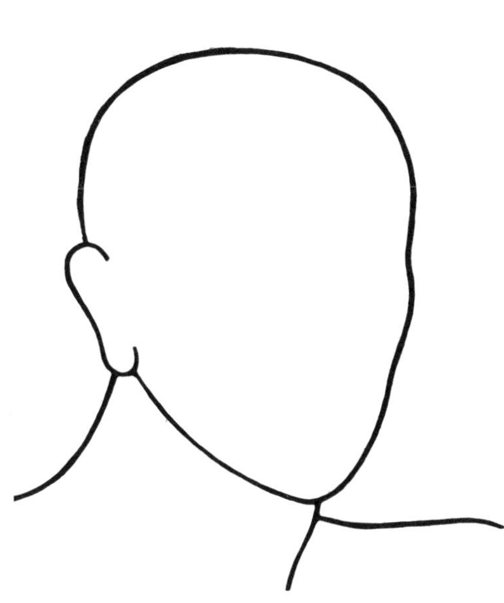

# 4

# LARC I and LARC II

For the first introduction to LARC, let's take a small problem. (After all, many of life's annoyances — little things that could use some creative input — are problems of no real significance.) The experimental problem presented here will be that old favorite: what uses can you find for a brick? But . . . what if thinking about a brick does not appeal to you? No matter. Though that is the problem under discussion here, you can learn LARC perfectly well using some other concept. You might, for instance, want to consider: what are some uses for (or different conceptions of) a *dog, money, land, silk, sports, freedom, fashion, wedding, paper, weapons?* If you want to use your own topic, just substitute it for the word brick in the exercises.

As a kind of test to see how you do *without* LARC, first see how many uses for a brick you can find on your *own*. Take a sheet (or sheets) of paper and list all the uses you can think of for a brick.

Uses for a Brick

1.
2.
3.
4.
5.
6.
7.
8.
9.
10.

If your brick uses run along the lines of "build something with bricks" or "throw a brick at your spouse," you *don't* get a gold star. Everyone will think of those things — for that's how we see bricks in our daily lives, in movies, stories, and cartoons. Now, let's use LARC for this "simple" problem.

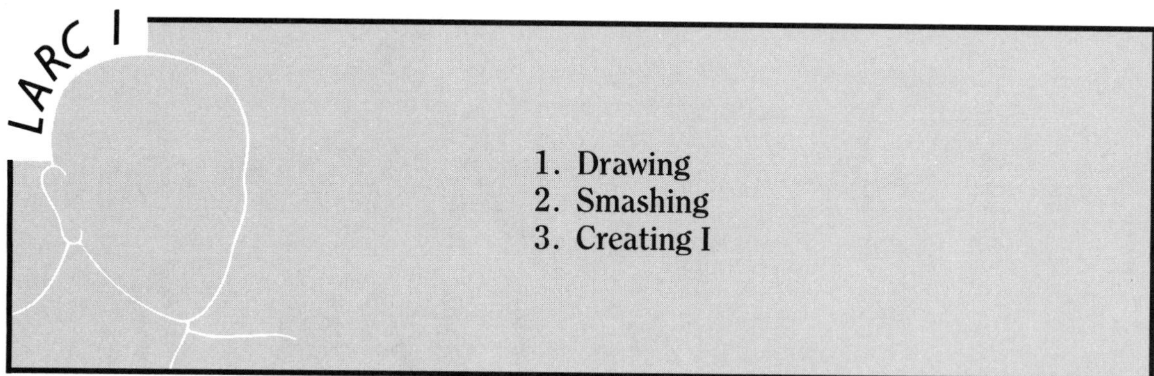


As you remember, the left brain is the *pattern user*, the right brain the *pattern seeker*. No doubt you also remember that once the left brain has a pattern to follow it does not want to change—this reluctance thwarting the pattern-seeking efforts of the right brain. It can be assumed, then, that when approaching any problem, people will have a firm, fixed, *old* pattern that needs to be "shaken up," broken down, if you will, so that the right brain can generate (seek) new patterns. In the problem, "What uses can you find for a brick?" "brick" is an established pattern for most of us. After all, we know what a brick is, what it does, what it is "good for." As result, it might be hard to think of many alternative uses for something as well "known" as a brick. The logical step to stimulate creative thinking, then, is to destroy a brick's "known" qualities, to free the right brain to do its work. First, the old structure or pattern of a brick (which is stored in the linguistic side of the brain) will be transformed into right-brain terms—pictorial images. Next, this pattern will be attacked with "Smashing questions." And finally, alternative patterns will be formed in the step called Creating I. So let's begin.

## Drawing

First, draw a picture of a brick.

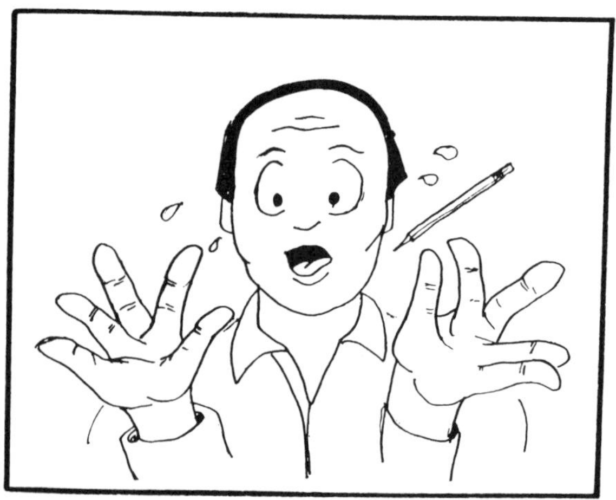

"What!" you cry. "Draw? I can't draw! My pictures look like those of a nine-year-old child. What if somebody should see me drawing little pictures? The men in the white coats would come and etc., etc., etc., etc." If you feel this way about drawing, it might help you to know that you are not alone. The response of our experimental subjects was often, "Do we *have* to draw pictures?" Yes. Sorry. And here's why. LARC is designed to cause shifts between the brains. It's known that the right brain is more pictorial than the left brain, so sketching pictures stimulates the right brain.

A number of other questions are always asked by experimental subjects. "What if someone *sees* me drawing...?" If you're worried about that, don't let them. Lock yourself in the bathroom if you must. "But how much detail should I attempt in my sketch?" It doesn't matter; since we're talking about a brick, however, you have time to draw it a number of ways: a profile, a three-dimensional object, an end of a brick, a bird's-eye view of a brick, etc. You may even like to write on it its *color*. The idea is to get a firm, mental picture of what the word brick means to you.

Now you may begin. Draw your picture (or pictures) of a brick on a sheet of paper. When you are satisfied with your brick (or bricks) continue with the next step.

## *Smashing*

The second stage of LARC I is called "Smashing." (Smashing combines the inventiveness of your right brain with the logic of your left brain.) You are now going to break down (smash) your brick into "fact-bits" by answering Smashing questions. Just how you go about this depends on the problem being investigated. For instance, four different lists of Smashing questions can be used — two "simple" lists that have only ten Smashing terms and two "complex" lists that contain twenty terms. As you might imagine, the simple lists of Smashing questions are for "easy" problems, the complex for "harder" problems. In addition, there are "passive" and "active" Smashing lists. Passive Smashing questions work best when smashing subjects or terms that have no independence of action, or cannot act on their own. A house is passive. So is a tree or a car. Conversely, active lists are for smashing terms that can control their actions — people, animals, organizations.

When beginning the Smashing step of LARC I, you want to determine whether or not your problem is simple or complex, then if the term to be smashed is active or passive. There are no absolute rules for selecting a Smashing list, however. Sometimes, in fact, it is hard to decide if the term you are smashing is active or passive. For instance, words such as nations, machines, or even organizations could be either active or passive. In these cases, you may want to try using both the active and passive lists to see what sorts of questions work best. There really is no way to be *wrong*, since if one Smashing list does not produce results, you can always switch to another. So try either the active or passive list; if it doesn't seem to be working, change to the other one.

Regarding a choice of simple or complex lists, it is almost always better to use the complex list. Use simple lists for only the most simple problems or when you have limited time to work on a problem.

The four lists of Smashing questions follow. Pause to read through them.

## Smashing Questions

### Passive

*Simple*

1. Types
2. Steps
3. Parts
4. Causes
5. When
6. Why
7. How
8. Things connected with
9. Sight images of
10. Products or results

*Complex*

1. Types
2. Steps
3. Parts
4. Causes
5. Synonyms
6. Who
7. What
8. When
9. Where
10. Why
11. How
12. Things connected with
13. Sight images of
14. Hearing images of
15. Emotions
16. Opposite
17. Touching images of
18. Characteristics
19. Products or results
20. Modes of operation

### Active

*Simple*

1. Abilities
2. Fear or threats
3. Goals and hopes
4. Strengths
5. Weaknesses
6. Types
7. Steps
8. Things connected with
9. Sight images of
10. Characteristics

*Complex*

1. Abilities
2. Fear or threats
3. Goals and hopes
4. Responsibilities
5. Interests
6. Likes
7. Dislikes
8. Strengths
9. Weaknesses
10. Types
11. Causes
12. Steps
13. How become
14. Who is
15. Where
16. When
17. Things connected with
18. Sight images of
19. Characteristics
20. Products or results

Returning to the "brick uses" problem, let's assume that you have decided to use the passive-complex list. (A brick is certainly passive — it can't be active.)

Listed below are the twenty Smashing words from the passive-complex list you will be using to smash the word brick into fact-bits. (*We have added a few sample fact-bits to the right of these Smashing words to give you an idea of some typical answers the Smashing words might suggest about the term brick.*)

### Smashing: brick

1. Types — *red, ceramic*
2. Steps — *clay, firing*
3. Parts —
4. Causes — *protection*
5. Synonyms —
6. Who —
7. What —
8. When — *culture gets advanced*
9. Where —
10. Why — *decorative*
11. How —
12. Things connected with — *buildings, walls, chimney*
13. Sight images of —
14. Hearing images of —
15. Emotions — *cold, angry, throw a brick*
16. Opposite —
17. Touching images of — *heavy*
18. Characteristics — *hard*
19. Products or results — *barrier, protective*
20. Modes of operation — *static, inflexible*

Consulting this list, you will find that one of the words is "types." Ask yourself if there are different types of bricks, then jot down all the kinds of bricks that come to mind. The list also gives you the phrase "sight images of." If you were working on another problem — "car" — you might list as "sight images of" — color, steering wheel, seat, radio, through the front window, door handle, tires, etc. You follow the same procedure for brick. (Note: some of the Smashing questions are designed to trigger the right brain, whereas others are more likely to tap the left.)

Try to list as many fact-bits beside each term as you can, but if you can think of nothing for a term, just leave the space blank. There is no one, right way to do this, though the more fact-bits you can generate, the better the creative results you can expect. Some terms may sound just the same to you. That's fine. They will *not* sound the same to other people. If you find yourself asking, "What does that term mean?" remember that what it means to you is all that's important. Along this line, you should be warned that some of the questions may sound strange to you when applied to brick ("who," for instance). That's O.K. Just interpret it in the way that seems most logical to you and write down any fact-bits that come to mind. You might interpret the question "who" as "Who would use bricks?" You are almost ready to begin, but first. . . .

## *Time Out*

Before you try the Smashing questions for the "brick uses" problem, you might like to see the fact-bits other people generated for completely different problems. Here are some examples:

### Examples of Answers to Smashing Questions

It is sometimes easier to generate your own fact-bits after looking at examples of fact-bits produced for different topics. A quick look at the subjects below might give you inspiration.

Topic: *Wedding*

4. Causes — *love, necessity, children, shotgun, social connection*
9. Where — *church, rose garden, hot-air balloon, home*
16. Opposite — *divorce, death (until death do you . . . ), living together — ending relationship*
19. Products or results — *children, divorce, richer or poorer, friendship, economic growth*
20. Modes of operation — *harmony, disharmony, pressure, tears (joy or sorrow of parent or jilted lover)*

Topic: *Dog*

2. Steps — *breeding, buy pet at shop, puppy, old dog, dog pan and dog house (get these for dog)*
6. Who — *owners: kids, lonely people, farmers, sheepherders, blind people; be reincarnated as a dog*
15. Emotions — *love, fear of neighbor's dog, loyalty, anger when it goes on rug, happiness in play*

(*Note:* the next examples for the term dog are questions from the active-complex list. As you can see, using different lists can be useful.)

4. Responsibilities — *dog: be friend, guard, protect, chase cats, track scent of animals; owner: take care of dog; love*
9. Weaknesses — *drool, bad doggy breath, short life, shedding, limited brain, bites people (law suit)*

Topic: *Car*

1. Types — *family, sports, railroad, streetcar, old, new, experimental, Ford, Volvo, etc., foreign*
14. Hearing images of — *loud, roar, backfire, purr, screech, crash, horn*
17. Touching images of — *smooth paint, hot in summer, cold in winter, hard steel, soft leather, feels like a friend, wet when washing car*
18. Characteristics — *shining, streamlined, powerful, dangerous, helpful, modern, problems*
19. Products or results — *transportation, pollution, economic clout, races, kills*

Topic: *Ambition*

3. Parts — *fame, wealth, power, control, corruption, ability*
5. Synonyms — *drive, lust, reaching, desire*
13. Sight images of — *clothing, cars, estates, horses, polo, big desk, crown, beautiful women*
16. Opposite — *defeat, humble, rags, shy*
17. Touching images of — *smooth silk, cold, elegant, offended (if someone who is rich is touched by a poor person)*

Have these examples helped? Let's hope so, for it's now time to try Smashing for yourself. Return to the list of Smashing questions on page 36. Copy the list on a piece of paper and then begin looking for fact-bits for brick. Spend about thirty seconds on each question. The sample fact-bit answers we included for some of the questions may assist you in getting started.

## Creating I

The next step, Creating I, is the final step in LARC I. The trick now is to turn information from the Smashing process into creative *solutions*. Do this by scrutinizing your "uses for a brick" page again; pore over every fact-bit to come up with some imaginative uses for a brick. For instance, you may have noted the color of the brick. Try to think of some way a brick could be used for its color. If a fact-bit for brick is "solid," try to find ways to use the solid qualities of a brick.

Are you ready? Start looking at your brick fact-bits one by one and write down uses for a brick that these bits suggest to you. (Put down bizarre uses as well, of course.)

You may also get good ideas from combining fact-bits. For example, if you got the fact-bit "protection" from the Smashing question "things connected with" and the fact-bit "designer" from the Smashing question "types," you might arrive at the idea of using some thin, yet stylish bricks as a new form of roofing — attractive, yet impervious to hail. Never mind, for the moment, what ideas will or will not work. The task at this point is to generate as many new patterns as possible. This is just an exercise; the idea is to create! Get another sheet of paper and begin.

| Uses for a Brick |
|---|
| 1. |
| 2. |
| 3. |
| 4. |
| 5. |
| 6. |
| 7. |
| 8. |
| 9. |
| 10. |

If you have decided to use only LARC I, you have now finished the "uses for a brick" problem. But should you wish to explore this (or any other) problem more fully, you can continue your search for creative ideas by moving on to LARC II.

## LARC II

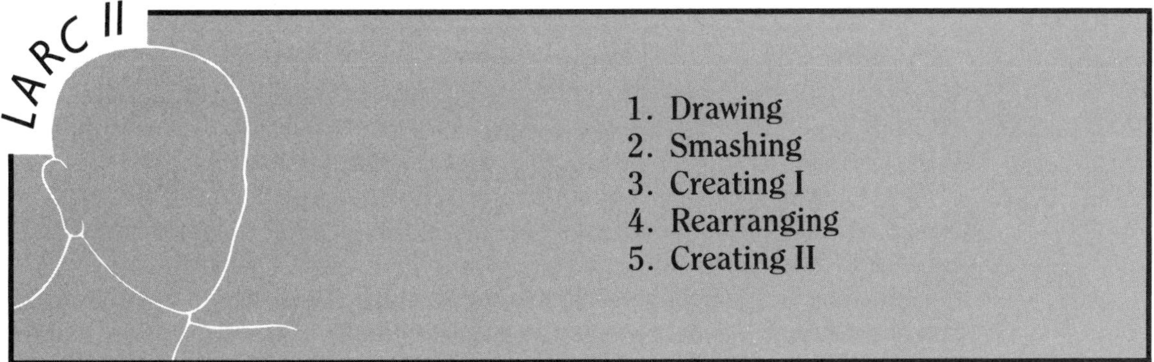

LARC I ended with Creating I, the step in which you generated creative ideas by the study and comparison of fact-bits. LARC II includes the same basic steps as LARC I (Drawing, Smashing, Creating I), but adds two steps (Rearranging and Creating II) that help in developing the creative idea. In brief, to use LARC II, follow the steps in LARC I, including the production of creative answers in Creating I. In the next stage, Rearranging, you do more work with fact-bits to put them into novel patterns from which a creative solution develops.

## *Rearranging*

To understand this step more fully, an analogy might be useful. When you were a child, you liked to work on jigsaw puzzles. After opening the box of a new puzzle, you would "tear up" the picture into its individual pieces. Then you fitted the parts together again and — surprise, surprise — had the very same picture with which you started. But let's suppose there were a new kind of jigsaw puzzle on the market in which every piece was shaped *exactly like* every other piece. The new puzzle would certainly be an easy one to work, though every time you put it together again, you would get an entirely different picture. True, each new picture would be a bit messy (modern artish), but you have to admit that each would be more creative than the old-style puzzle with which you keep rebuilding the same picture over and over.

In a similar manner, you drew a brick, then smashed it into hardly recognizable fact-bits. Now, much like the new type of jigsaw puzzle, you will *rearrange* your brick any way you want, creating a new picture of it. This stage of Rearranging is called a "Group." Looking at the fact-bits you have generated by smashing your brick, you will notice that some fall into patterns or groups. For instance, if you were working on a problem on "war," some of your fact-bits might be:

3. Parts — *treaties, nations, bombs go off, cook's pans rattle, sergeants shouting*
4. Causes — *radical ideas, territory*
9. Sight images of — *soldiers, nurses, shells, buddies, having a bullet wound*
10. Products or results — *death, destruction, being separated from family*

After looking at the fact-bits, someone might put them in the following Groups:

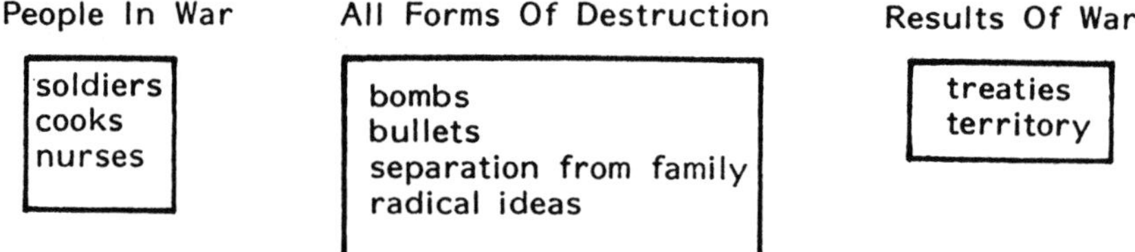


Note that each Group is labeled — "People in War," "All Forms of Destruction," "Results of War."

In Rearranging, your job is to find as many Groups as you can for your fact-bits. Be sure to label each Group according to its subject. For instance, just from the fact-bits provided as examples, the following Groups might be formed:

| Things That Would Make A Loud Noise If They Fell | Moods | Ways To Stop A Bullet |
|---|---|---|
| heavy things | hard | barrier |
| chimneys | angry | wall |
| walls | cold | hard things |
| buildings | heavy | |

Now find and label Groups from your brick fact-bits. Use as many Groups as you need. Naturally, the more Groups you can find, the better. When finished, continue reading.

### *Creating II*

Using the Groups from Rearranging, develop additional solutions to the "brick uses" problem. Look at your Groups and see if their *titles* give you any ideas about brick usage, or if the fact-bits within the Groups suggest other ways a brick could be of service. (Of course, you can combine the titles of a Group with any of the fact-bits to get an idea.) Write any new uses on the "uses for a brick" page, using more paper if necessary.

## *How Did You Do?*

You may now want to compare your "uses for a brick" answers that were generated using LARC I and II with those you thought of all by yourself on page 33. Did LARC I and II help? (Note: the more you experiment with LARC, the more comfortable you will become with it; the easier LARC gets for you, the more really creative ideas you will come up with!)

## *How Others Did*

Just for fun, you might like to compare the way you worked the "uses for a brick" problem with the way it was handled by several of our *best* experimental subjects, who were working *together* on the problem. Their work follows. Note particularly the "uses" pages, where the subjects' answers are recorded, complete with discussions of how the solutions were generated.

*Brick*

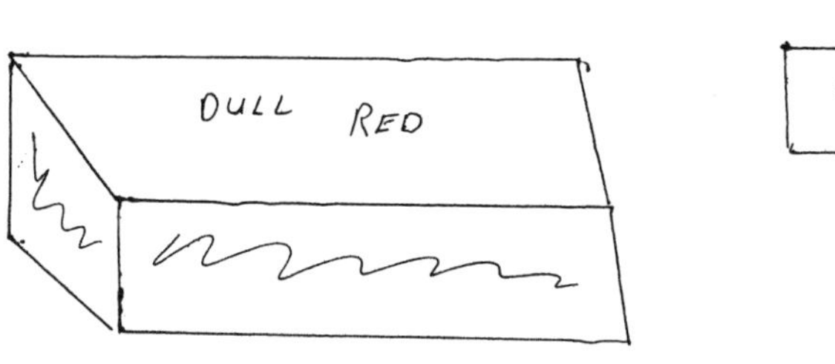


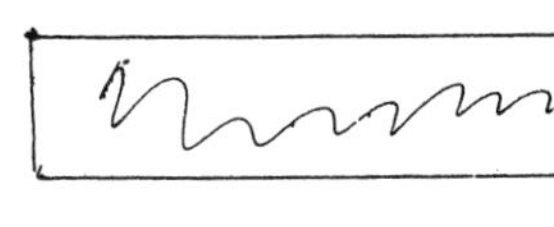

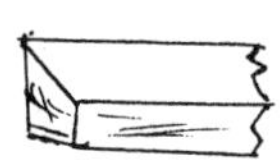

## *Sample Answers*
## *Smashing: brick*

1. Types — *fire bricks, sun-dried, kiln-dried, glazed, small, large, written on*
2. Steps — *clay and water, mud, oven, fire, cool, build with (brick steps)*
3. Parts — *clay, straw, water, fire to bake them, paint, glaze, ceramic (Assyrian baked walls, lions, funny animals on them), break them in half*
4. Causes — *need to stay out of wind, cold, wet; no good stone, few trees, lots of clay*
5. Synonyms — *tablet, building block*
6. Who — *Who owns it? Who makes it? Who needs it? Who has it thrown at him? Who is called a brick? comments on early history*
7. What — *building material; clay, sun-dried with straw; cuneiform writing on early Sumerian bricks; artificial bricks for fireplaces, for writing, Sumerians*
8. When — *early Sumerians in history, lack good stone; all through history; arch, dome, fireproofing, poor insulation, when need solid construction*
9. Where — *private buildings, public, defense fort, for sign, at brickyard, displays at home shows, fireplaces, Sumerian temples*
10. Why — *need solid construction, cheap to build with, rain doesn't get through, kiln-dried bricks, good for compression (hold lot of weight); can't see through them, privacy, fences, hide behind in war*
11. How — *make them in brick molds, fire them in oven, come in many sizes, some decorative*
12. Things connected with — *houses, factories, someone throwing one, mortar, historical corner boxes, paint*
13. Sight images of — *dull red, rectangle, sharp edges, sharp corners, rough surfaces, could be chips off it, broken in half, with rugged break, cut into pieces, part of a wall; can paint them many colors; sinking in water*
14. Hearing images of — *sound it makes when thrown: against glass, other brick, ground; a thud, popping in oven, rain hitting, breaking, scratching against it or mortar slapped against it, splash in water*
15. Emotions — *not much personality, solid, feel good when it's holding up the house*
16. Opposite — *anything soft, anything smooth, anything porous, anything light*
17. Touching images of — *could feel rough or smooth, depends on coarseness of your fingers, sharp edges and corners, very rough when broken, feels heavy*
18. Characteristics — *rough or smooth, many colors, sharp edges, heavy, solid, dull in color, solid construction, holds up weight, cheap, thick, stores heat, hard, clumsy, breakable*
19. Products or results — *buildings, employment*
20. Modes of operation — *build them by hand, and build buildings out of them by hand; trowel, mortar, work clothes, hard-toed shoes*

## *Groups*

**Kinds Of Bricks**

fancy, glazed
sun-dried
kiln-dried
different sizes
different clays

**How Made**

water
straw
clay
brick mold
oven
cooled

**Owners**

makers
middlemen
home owners
city in street
children to play with
dogs -- their houses

**Forms Of Construction**

post and lintel
arch
dome
solid for defense
for privacy
fireplace--won't burn
use artificial bricks--
look good but cheap
outhouse

**Surfaces**

smooth glaze
regular semi-rough
broken into jagged pieces
ground up

**Sounds When Thrown**

crash against hard surface
breaking glass
hitting ground-thud
hitting water-splash
still hitting air-hiss

**As Weapon**

throw at enemy
hit him
he throws it back
hits you

**Factory**

smokestack
walls
foundation

**Who Owns It**

king--capital city
noble--villa
commoner--house
brickmaker

**Quality Of Brick**

kiln-dried with glaze
kiln-dried
sun-dried

**Size Of Buildings**

fortifications
public buildings
private homes
outhouse
dollhouse

**Building**

level area
brick
mortar on top
another brick
stagger the bricks
for strength
half-brick to finish line

**How Destroyed**

chipped
eroded by weather
broken
ground to dust

**Thrown Brick**

pick up, through window
hit dog, owner curses
run away

**Weight**

large brick
small brick
piece of brick
brick dust

**Archeology**

dig
find brick
clean
deciphered writing
understand culture
in museum

**Building With Brick**

foundation
wall
fireplace
privacy fence
sidewalk

## *Sample Answers*
## *Uses for a Brick*

1. Put some bricks in the back of the toilet to take up space so less water would be used when flushing. This saves on high water bills when there is a water shortage.

*Getting the Answer:* "We got this answer by putting together some of the fact-bits we had for several Smashing questions. We noticed that we had the term 'solid construction' under 'why' and 'when.' We were talking about when you could use something that was solid when we also noticed the fact-bit 'sinking in water,' which we had under 'sight images of.' Somebody said as a sort of joke that we could use bricks to fill up a pond. Of course, that didn't seem very helpful. But when we saw the term 'cheap' also under 'why,' it suddenly hit us that there was a practical way to use sinking bricks that would actually make things cheaper for a family. This was, of course, our answer about the bricks and the toilet tank."

2. Scratch on bricks historical events that you want to last a long time. This would be helpful to archeologists.

*Getting the Answer:* "We got this answer by looking at the Group labeled 'Archeology.' The words we had inside this Group all led us to think of history, and the term 'writing' got us thinking that if you could write on bricks they would be a long-lasting record that archeologists might dig up thousands of years in the future. Sumerians did this on clay bricks."

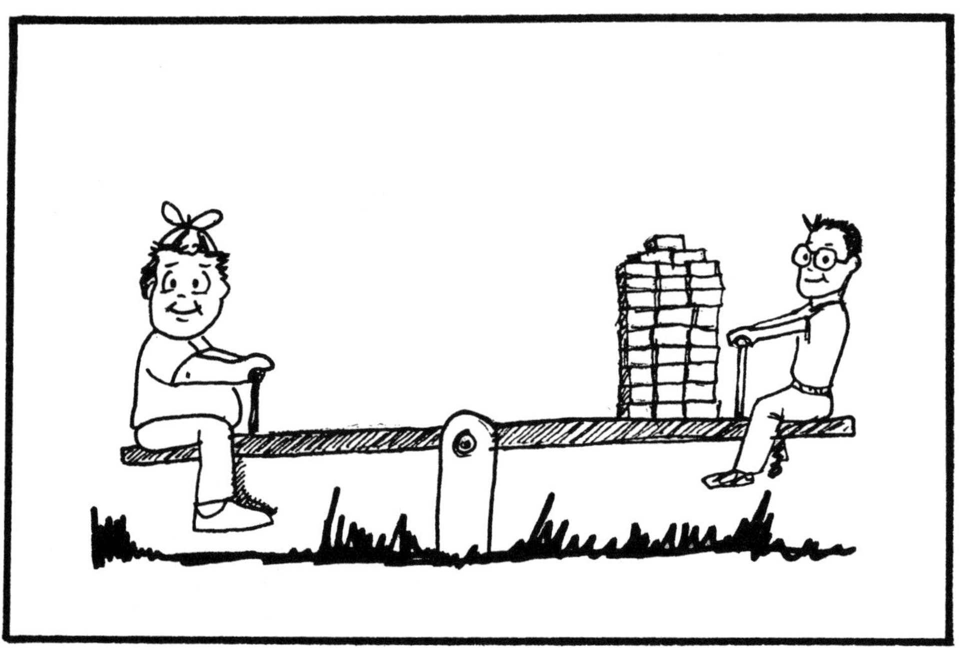

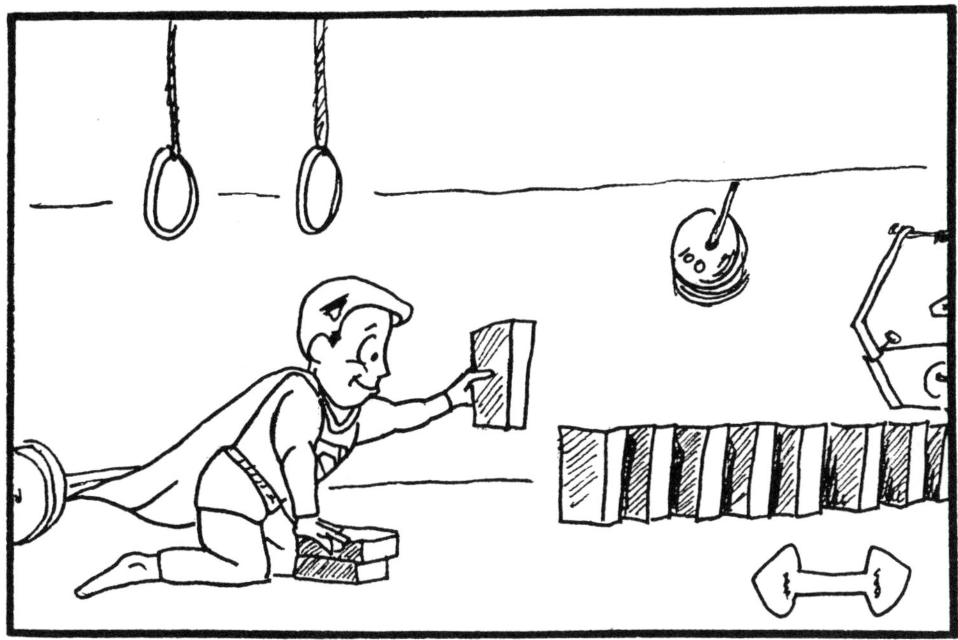


*Super baby's first domino set.*

3. Bricks could be used as a crude but very permanent monetary system. You could even break them in half, the parts making change. This might be necessary after a major disaster like an atomic war, which would disrupt the cultures of the world.

*Getting the Answer:* "Our first idea that led to this solution came when we looked at the Group we labeled 'Who Owns It.' In this case, it was really just the title of the Group that got us going. The idea of ownership obviously made us think of buying things — of money. We also noticed from our fact-bits that we had gotten a number of references of bricks being used for building, even in ancient times. One person said that to be used as building materials, bricks generally had to be the same size and shape. It was then that we first thought of using bricks for money. After all, if they are the same size, it would give a common unit. Finally, the idea that this could be useful after a major disaster came from our appreciation of how hard it was to destroy bricks. This we got from another Group we labeled 'How Destroyed.' Communications between nations would be wiped out. But bricks are harder to destroy than regular money, and besides, everyone knows what bricks are, and that would solve some communication problems."

4. Use a brick to turn on the light switch to keep from being shocked when standing in water in the basement.

*Getting the Answer:* "The way we got this answer was really odd. It started when we were talking about how bricks hold heat (fact-bit from our 'characteristics' question). Someone was talking about how the bricks on the inside of his fireplace were meant to hold heat. Then one of us said he didn't have a fireplace, that he heated with electricity, that bricks wouldn't help with this since they don't conduct electricity. That's when we got the idea that this disadvantage of bricks could really be an advantage sometimes when dealing with electricity."

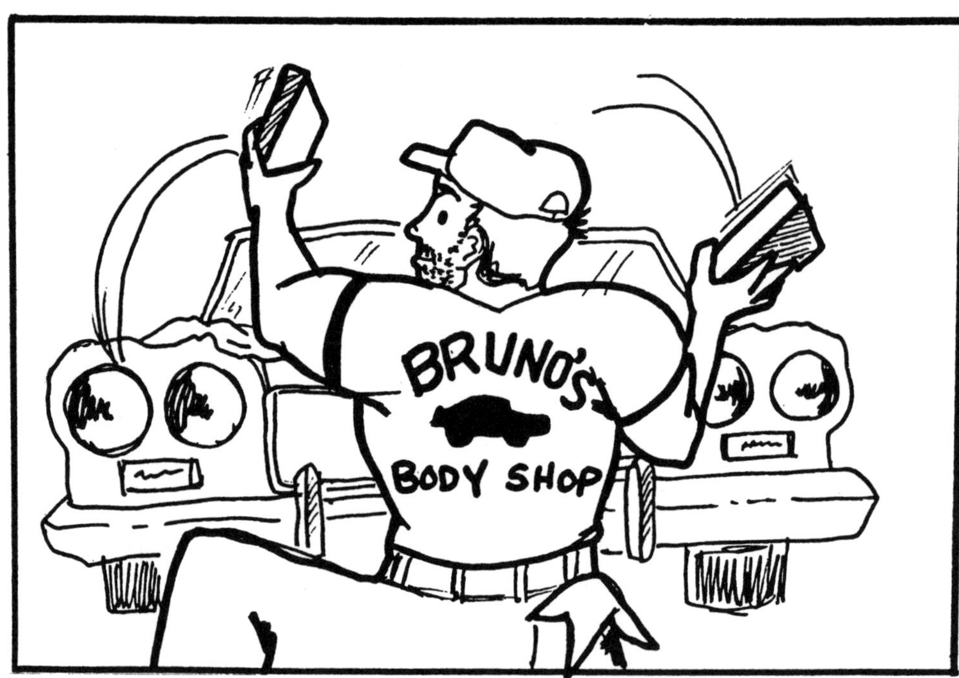


*Drumming up business.*

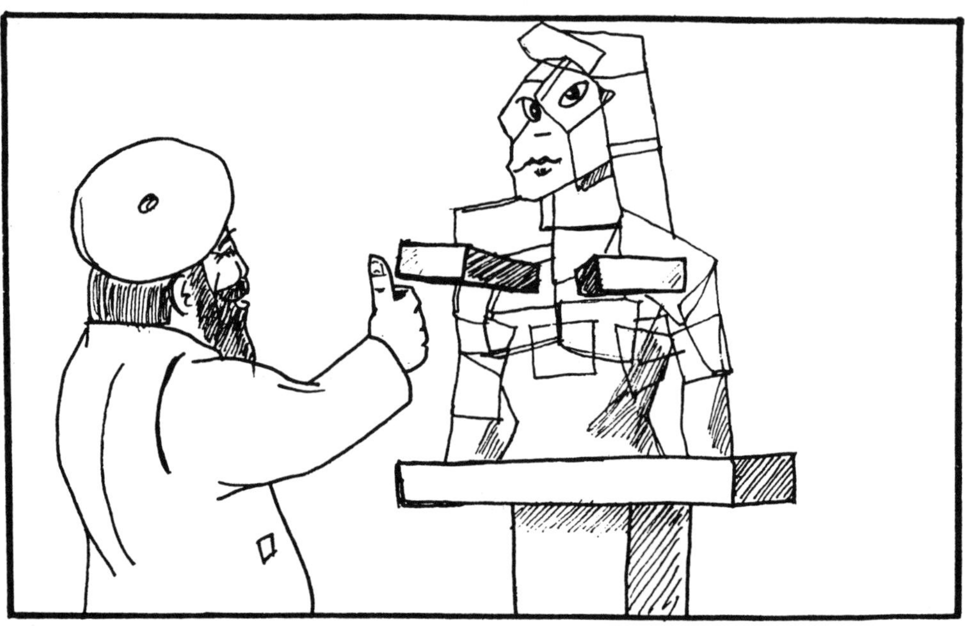

## Summary

From looking at some of the preceding examples, you can see that "breakthrough" ideas don't always come immediately. In fact, when examining seemingly irrelevant fact-bits and Groups, it often takes a little time to generate a creative idea. LARC helps break down a fixed concept by Smashing, then gives the right brain a chance to shuffle the resultant fact-bits into new patterns.

These solutions were given not only to show several answers from some of our better subjects, but also to illustrate how these answers were formulated. A quick review shows that subjects found their solutions in a wide variety of ways, including: (1) looking at an isolated fact-bit; (2) direct comparison of two or more fact-bits; (3) forming an answer from the terms within a Group; (4) getting an answer from just the title of a Group; (5) comparing two or more Groups for a solution; (6) getting an answer from a combination of fact-bits *and* Groups! The combinations are legion.

LARC stimulates a number of ideas and concepts about a topic that serve as the mix from which the right brain can generate a host of patterns. The more right-brain activity, the better chance the left brain has to select an answer that will work. The key is just to get the process started. Break down the existing pattern a person already has of a concept, and the "broken" pattern of fact-bits will lead to creative thinking.

Obviously, some of our subjects' answers produced for the "brick uses" problem may not be practical, but then again, it was merely an exercise.

Of course, there is one suggestion that just might save your life — using a brick to turn on a light when your feet are in water! A brick might not be handy at

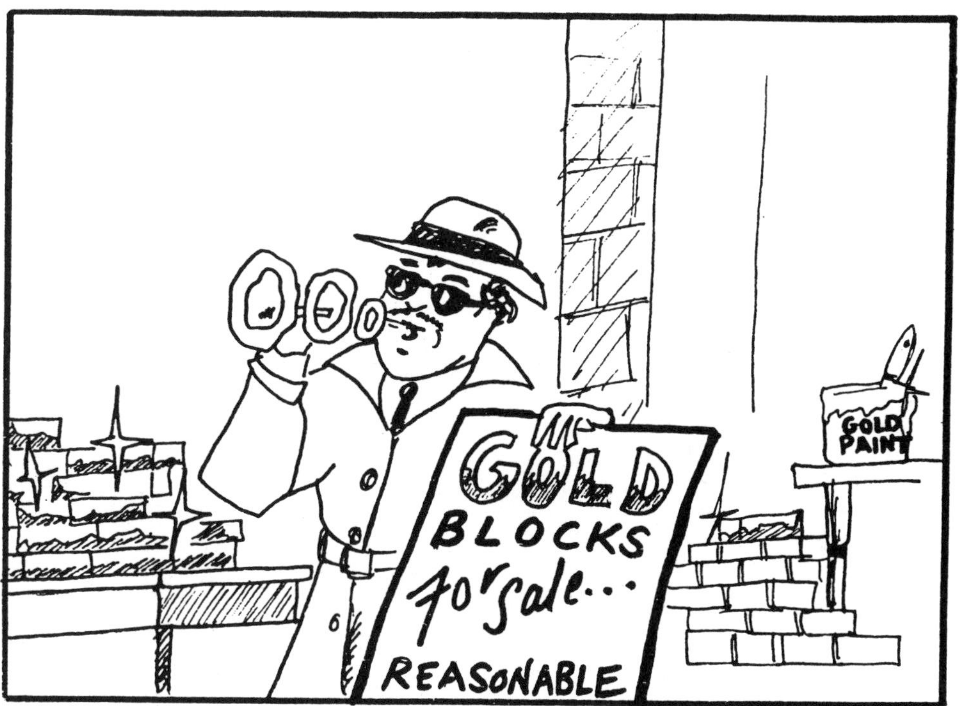


*The best* possible *use of a brick.*

such a time, but one creative thought tends to lead to another — for instance, finding a dry broom handle or a piece of rolled-up paper with which to flip the light switch.

Once more, though, the point of using LARC is to help generate creativity; it gives you something to work with when you need that inventive solution. Then, too, remember that all you have been doing so far is learning to work LARC. Think how exciting this will become when you first start solving problems that mean something to you!

## For All Practical Purposes

You will be glad to know that what you have learned to do so far (LARC I and II) is all you will ever need to stimulate the production of many creative solutions. But, as indicated in chapter 3, some problems are more complex, more stubborn, and will take additional effort before inventive solutions make themselves evident.

So, to repeat, first try LARC I to see if it gives you the answer you wish. If nothing usable surfaces, continue with LARC II. Still not satisfied? Don't worry. LARC III and IV follow.

A final and happy thought is that the more practice a person has with LARC, the more likely that person will be to develop the ability to make the necessary left-right brain switches . . . automatically! If that happens, then the individual will become like the star athlete who "just naturally" moves with grace and precision or, for that matter, the "naturally creative" person whose ideas just pop up out of the blue. As with the athlete, the key is *practice*, in this case practice in making the right-left brain switches with LARC. With a little time, most people should find themselves becoming more naturally creative, needing less time to find the inventive solutions they seek.

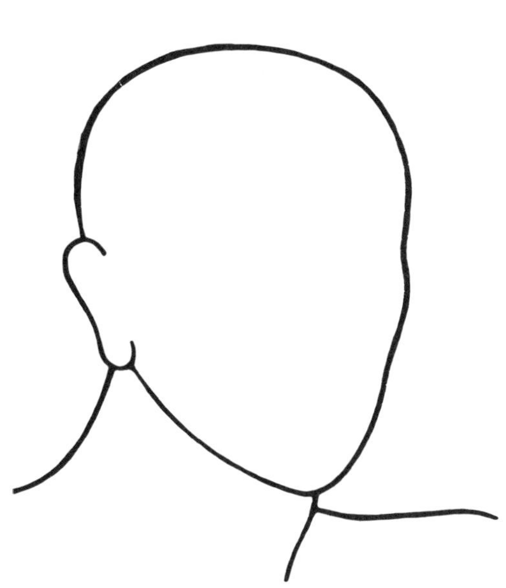

# 5 Extended Applications and LARC III

The first example of LARC dealt with a single pattern (a brick) that had to be broken down before it could be explored creatively. A person often has a simple problem involving one major word or pattern (for example, How will I spend my *vacation*?), but in other cases, a creative solution connecting two or more terms or patterns is required (How can I combine my roles as *wife* and *worker*? or What Christmas present can I buy that will please both Uncle *James* and Aunt *Sally*?).

LARC will work for these more complex problems also. Remember, finding a connection or pattern between two or more distinct terms is a natural process for the right brain. All that most people need is a system that triggers this process.

But . . . do you still doubt your right brain's ability to find new patterns? If so, all you must do, oh skeptic, is try the following exercise. . . . Then repent!

## Your Right Brain in Action—An Exercise

Let's try to add some support to the assertion that the right brain is naturally creative, that it just *naturally* finds new patterns, by giving you a chance to see how *your own* right brain can produce novel patterns. In the following experiment, you will be given clues, the majority of which point to a well-known literary work. (A few of them, which do not fit the pattern at all, are ruses to throw you off the track. You wouldn't be impressed with your right brain's creative prowess if this were *too* easy, now would you?) Look at the list until you think you can guess the work, success in doing so a demonstration of your right brain's talent for creating a pattern from a variety of data. Here are some clues to a work of literature:

tragic
automobile
family hatred
horses
ancestors
boy and girl
romantic love
yellow
death
suicide

After you think you have the answer, continue reading.

"Horses," "automobile," and "yellow" don't belong; the rest of the words fit the pattern of *Romeo and Juliet* by Shakespeare. If you thought of *Romeo and Juliet*, and eighty-five percent of people taking this test do, can you remember how that answer "popped" into your mind? Is it possible it came to you, not as the words "Romeo and Juliet," but first as a mental picture — the famous balcony scene, perhaps? Many people say they first *saw a picture* of the balcony scene before thinking of the words for that picture. This experience demonstrates that the creative right brain is pictorial, understands in the form of pictures. (You might be interested to know that Einstein always claimed that solutions came to him in pictures.) As for finding the *Romeo and Juliet* pattern, this feat is little short of amazing (even though it may not seem so since the right brain performs this kind of "magic" all the time). Starting with only a few words, some of them misleading, your right brain shifted the various words around, forming patterns until it arrived at an answer that the left brain deemed appropriate. Impressive, don't you think?

Of course, you may have gotten a completely different pattern from this word list. One subject said he thought the pattern was the television program, "Dallas"; several words in the list fit that mold as well. The right brain may discover any number of inventive combinations — as long as the left brain will *let* it. (If you didn't find a pattern in this list, it's all right. It doesn't mean anything about whether or not you can *learn* to be creative.)

## Creative Courage

The fact that you're still reading shows you're serious about developing creativity. Good — though it's only fair to warn you that inventive people run special risks. One of them is getting enthused by novel ideas! Before you're through with the book, you will be generating many exciting concepts of your own. Please remember that you're new at this and so should exercise caution in such areas as buying stock, mixing chemicals, testing experimental hang gliders, and believing government reports about the safety of breathing radioactive dust. Seriously, about the only harm you will suffer by improving your imaginative powers is having your GREAT IDEAS ridiculed as "impractical." At such times, consider that one of the finest minds of all time, Leonardo da Vinci, couldn't make his flying machine fly. Remember, too, that da Vinci's fame today, far from being damaged by this failure, has been enhanced by his having the foresight and courage to make the attempt!

## The More Difficult or Multi-sided Problem

Now that you are emboldened by da Vinci's example, it's time for a second run through LARC, this time with a "multi-sided" problem. In addition, LARC III will be introduced, though you have already learned its basic parts – Drawing, Smashing, Creating I, Rearranging, and Creating II. And here is your multi-sided problem:

Find the similarities between "*school*" and "*island.*"

"What?" you say. "That's the dumbest thing I ever heard. There is *nothing* the same about *school* and *island*, and who cares, anyway?" Ah, ah, ah. Careful! You don't want to join the people loitering around Leonardo's airplane, kicking the tires and proclaiming it will never get off the ground because God didn't intend men to fly.

Anyway, you never know when comparing seemingly unrelated entities will produce positive results. Someone combined chocolate and peanut butter – ugh! – and came up with Reese's Peanut-butter Cups. Another person put the unwanted explosive potential of cleaning fluid (gasoline) together with metal parts to invent the first practical internal-combustion engine. Gutenberg united a wine press, black paint, tin, lead, and antimony to make *printing* possible.

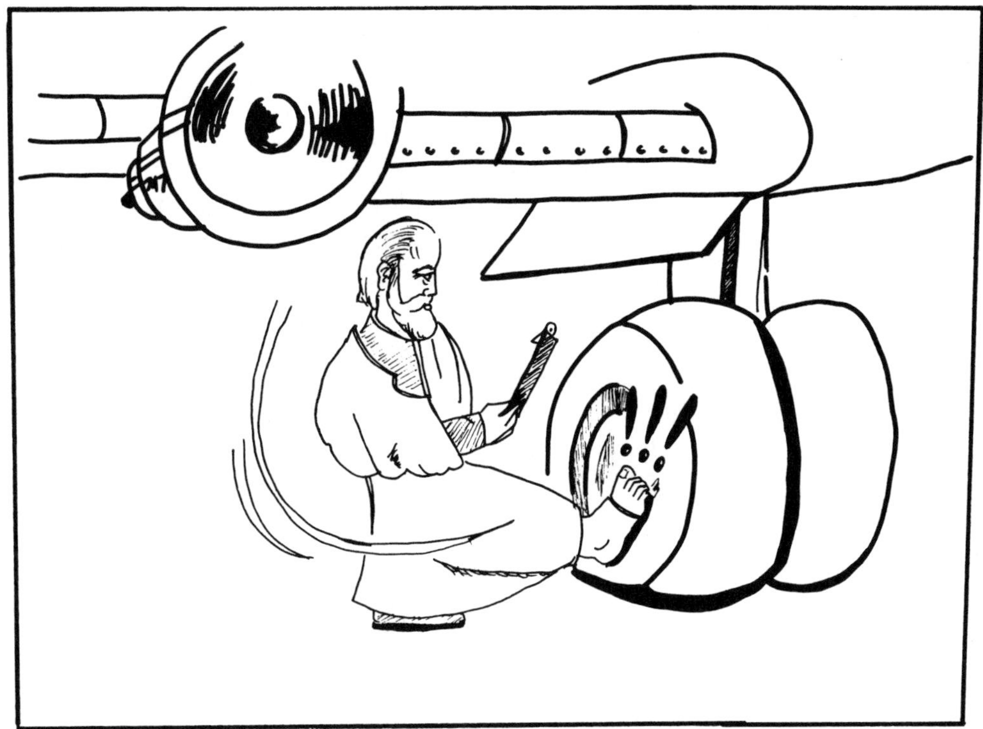

(Practically speaking, you're right, of course, that no one wants to find similarities between school and island, but you have to admit that any resemblances that can be discovered will certainly be *creative*.) An additional benefit of using this particular problem is that you have not heard it discussed, so any similarities you find will be the result of your own inventiveness. And again, odd as it sounds, we've found this problem to be a good teaching device.

But . . . before we continue, let's see what you can do without LARC. Remember, the problem is: Find the similarities between school and island. First list everything you can think of that's the same about school and island; work on it for as long as you wish.

Similarities between
School and Island

1.
2.
3.
4.
5.
6.
7.
8.
9.
10.

We don't know what *you* listed, but an experimental subject could think of only one connection at this stage of the process:

They both are limited: one by a fence, the other by the sea.

That's not bad. (If you were an artist getting ready to paint a school or an island that concept might even be of value to you.) But it's only one resemblance, after all.

Was your experience the same? Did you think and think and come up with only a few similarities? Why? From what we know of the mind, your creative right brain was simply bubbling with "fun" connections, many of them wild, even crazy—most, if not all, of them batted back by a left brain that refused even to consider such "silly" thoughts. LARC helps you combat this lack of communication between the "brains," to let more of these wild, creative ideas flow from your right brain to your left, where you can "get to them." "But," you ask, "won't many of these right brain ideas—like dreams—be absurd?" No doubt they will. But even the most fanciful idea may be modified into something useful, making it better to have a "dumb" idea than "no" idea.

So let's begin the "school and island" problem using (for now) LARC I.

## LARC I

### *Drawing*

As we learned in chapter 3, the first step of LARC is drawing. Draw school and island.

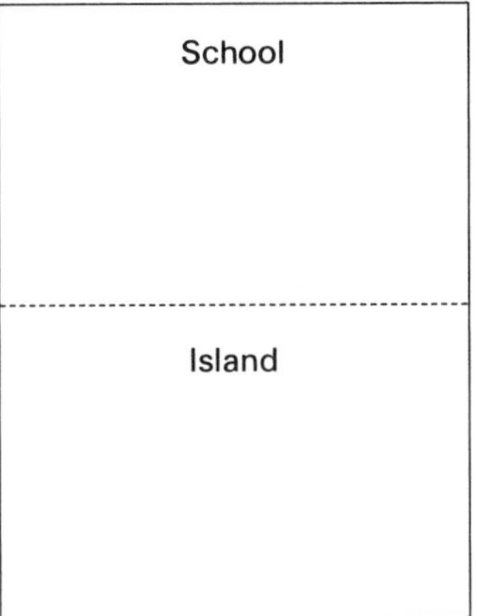


In case you're interested, here are some other people's pictures of school and island.

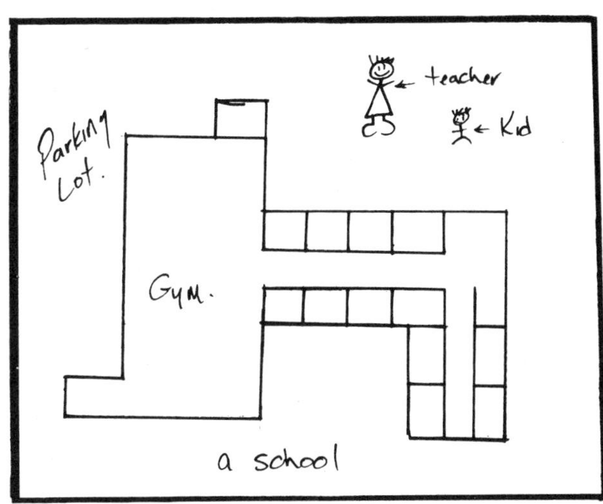


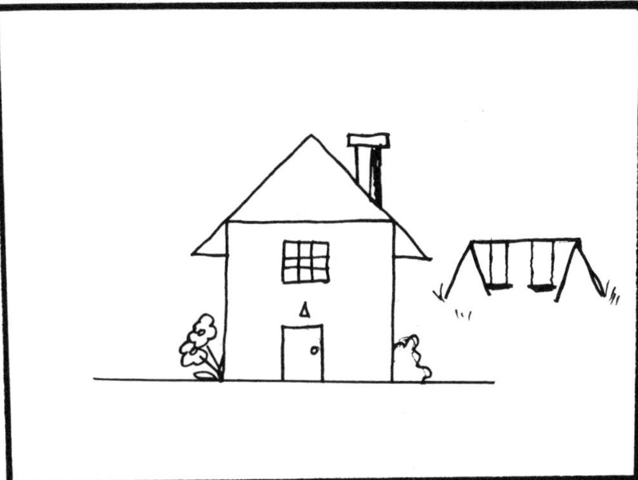

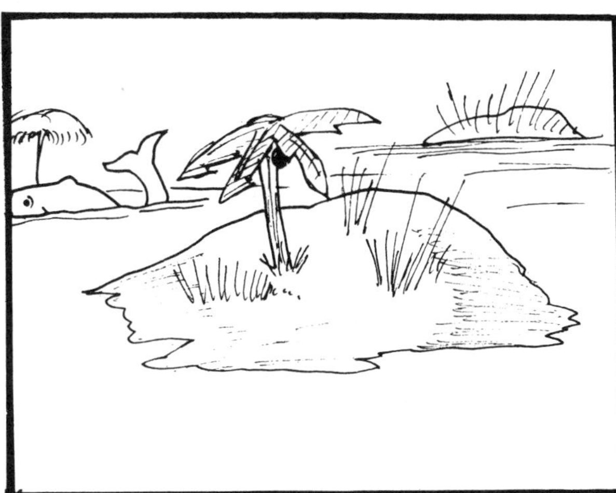

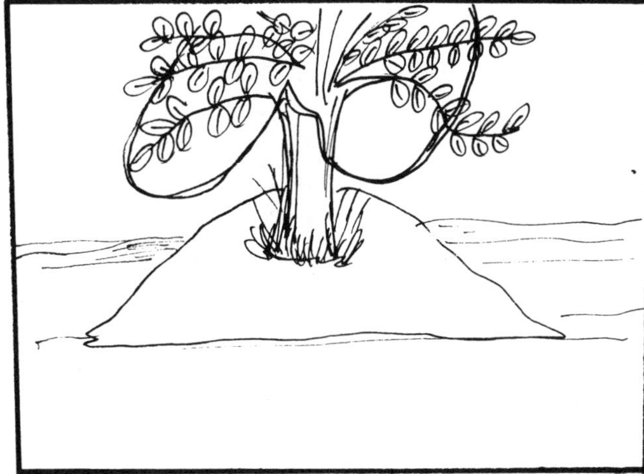

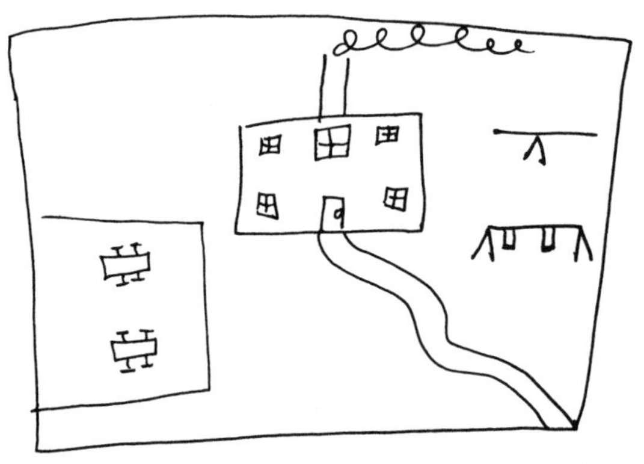

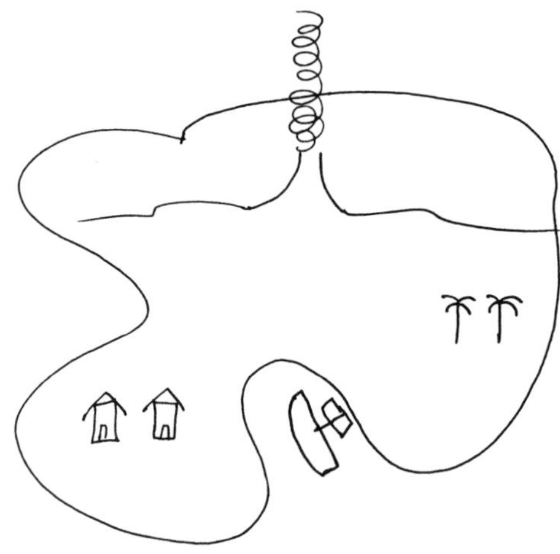

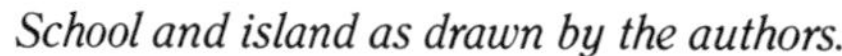

*School and island as drawn by the authors.*

## Smashing

Next, as in the "uses for a brick" problem, smash the pictures of school and island into fact-bits. We recommend, again, the use of the complex list for Smashing. Since school and island are rather passive, use the passive-complex list of Smashing words and phrases. Look at your picture of school for help, but don't be limited by it. Put down any fact-bit that comes to mind (whether or not it is in the picture). Remember, spend no longer than thirty seconds on each of the Smashing terms. (To get started, you *could* peek at some sample answers on page 55.)

List the smashing terms below on a sheet of paper. Write your answers there; use as many sheets as you need.

### Smashing: school

1. Types
2. Steps
3. Parts
4. Causes
5. Synonyms
6. Who
7. What
8. When
9. Where
10. Why
11. How
12. Things connected with
13. Sight images of
14. Hearing images of
15. Emotions
16. Opposite
17. Touching images of
18. Characteristics
19. Products or results
20. Modes of operation

When finished, continue.

That wasn't too bad, was it? Let's hope not because — you guessed it — you are now to do the same with island, looking at your picture of island for help. Don't be limited by your picture, though. Put down any fact-bit about island your brain churns out. The more bits, the better. Limit yourself to thirty seconds per Smashing term. (Some sample answers are on page 56.) Again, copy the smashing terms below and write your answers.

### *Smashing: island*

1. Types
2. Steps
3. Parts
4. Causes
5. Synonyms
6. Who
7. What
8. When
9. Where
10. Why
11. How
12. Things connected with
13. Sight images of
14. Hearing images of
15. Emotions
16. Opposite
17. Touching images of
18. Characteristics
19. Products or results
20. Modes of operation

When finished, continue.

A few terms are listed below to satisfy your curiosity about what other people got for fact-bits.

### *Smashing: school*

3. Parts—*brick, mortar, minds*
4. Causes—*compulsory, parents, curiosity, friends*
10. Why—*man is curious . . . and snobbish*
17. Touching images of—*no touching (a few punches on the playground)*

### *Smashing: island*

3. Parts—*sand, trees, wind, sea (the sea is the most important one, "y'sea")*
4. Causes—*volcanoes, pressure, heat, atmosphere*
10. Why—*inadequacies of the sea*
17. Touching images of—*slithering, bland sand through the fingers — warm, warm, warm*

Since multi-sided problems take (this will not come as a great revelation to you) *twice* as long as simple problems, it is time for you to rest. There are two reasons for this. In the first place, a fresh mind functions better than a tired one, and in the second, creative thoughts come more readily after a break. Remember that Archimedes got his idea about specific gravity while relaxing at the bathhouse; the same experience of creation following rest was true for Coleridge, Kekulé, Howe, and many others. The creativity researcher, Graham Wallas, called this stage Incubation, you will remember. Take at least a half hour to rest.

## *Creating I*

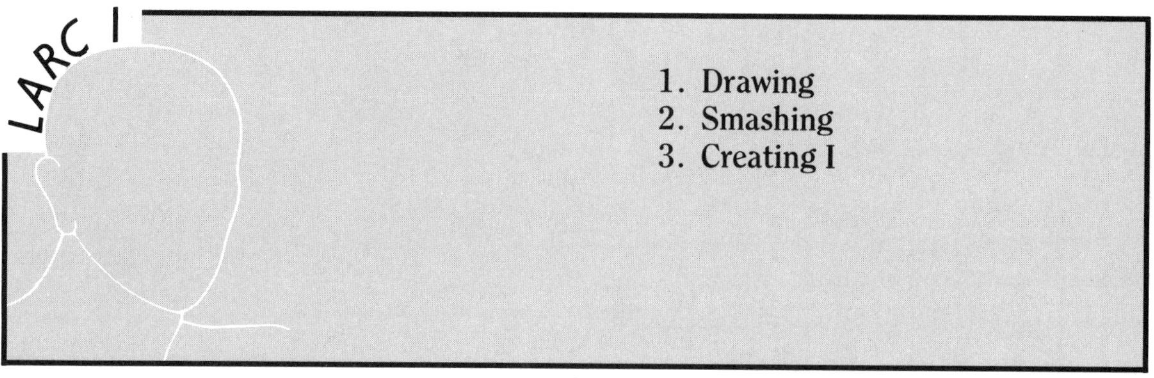


If you are using only LARC I, all that remains is Creating I, looking for ideas by matching fact-bits from school with those from island. If you are working through this sample problem, go ahead and complete Creating I now. How many similarities can you find between school and island just by comparing fact-bits? You may be surprised! Write down your answers on a sheet of paper.

| Similarities Between School and Island |
|---|
| 1. |
| 2. |
| 3. |
| 4. |
| 5. |
| 6. |
| 7. |
| 8. |
| 9. |
| 10. |

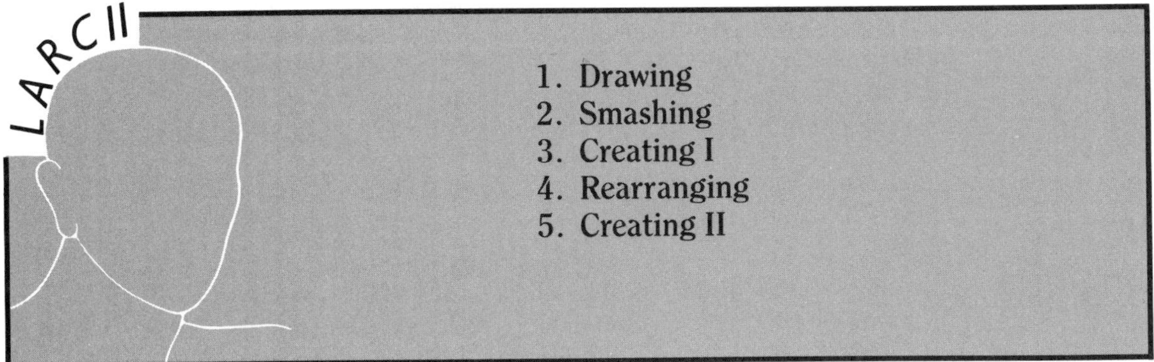


If you were to continue with LARC II, you would add the steps Rearranging and Creating II. But don't do this now because with this example of school and island you will learn the next version of LARC — LARC III.

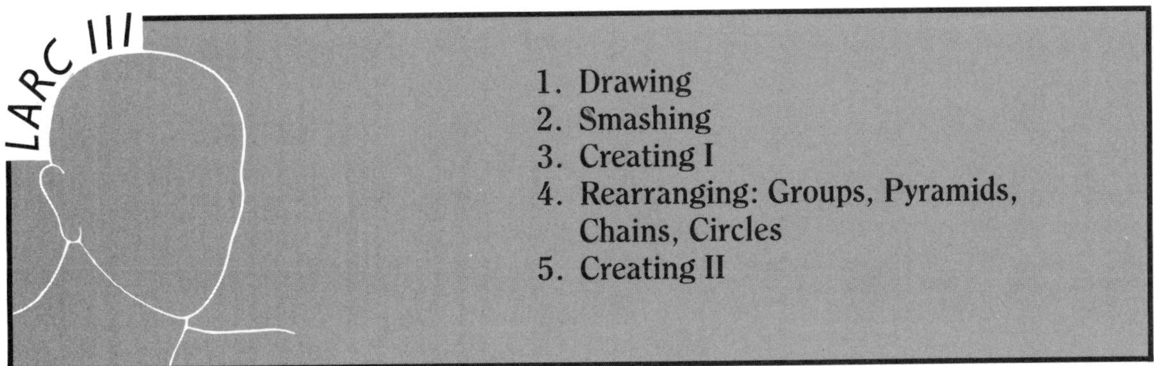


LARC III has the same steps as LARC II, but more parts are added to the Rearranging stage. Before discussing these, let's review what you have already learned about Rearranging.

## *Rearranging: Review*

After Smashing and Creating I, (examining each fact-bit for its possible creative potential), comes *Rearranging*. In the "uses for a brick" problem, the fact-bits with something in common were arranged in Groups. You need to do this again. Take a piece of paper and write down any Groups you find for school. Give each Group a title indicating just what kinds of fact-bits are included. Make as many Groups as you can. Here is an example:

People At School

principal
students
teachers
janitors
visitors

If you were working with LARC II, you would now go to the step Creating II (after making Groups for island, of course) and look for more creative ideas generated by your work with Groups. But let's assume that you wanted to look at the problem in greater depth. Then you would continue with LARC III.

## LARC III — Rearranging

It is now time to introduce three additional tools for *Rearranging*. In LARC III, Rearranging includes not only Groups, but also Rearranging tools called "Pyramids," "Chains," and "Circles." Pyramids, Chains, and Circles are just additional ways to arrange fact-bits into new patterns. So to continue with Rearranging in LARC III, let us discuss the concept of the Pyramid.

### Pyramid

Another word for Pyramid might be hierarchy, which means things placed in an order from top to bottom.

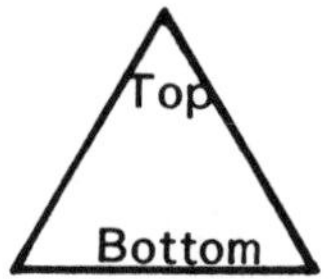


After constructing Groups, search the fact-bits for items that fall into an order that can be arranged in a Pyramid. Such an order might be top to bottom, high to low, strong to weak, noisy to quiet—or any other order that occurs to you.

Let's take some examples. Suppose you've been working not on school and island but on some other problem that has caused you to generate the following fact-bits:

lawn mower
quasar
Christmas, Easter, my birthday
moon
state officials, local officials
president, senators
tank, car, black hole
tractor, blender, county officials
happiness, sadness
workers
sun, lemons, coke

Do any of these fact-bits seem to "go together"? Could you arrange any of them in some Pyramidal shape, in some hierarchy from top to bottom? Take a minute to study these fact-bits—it's good practice. When finished, continue reading for some examples of Pyramids using these sample fact-bits.

You may have noticed several political leaders listed as fact-bits. They are "county officials," "local officials," "state officials," "president," and "senators." Can you arrange these officials into a Pyramid? How about the following Pyramid?

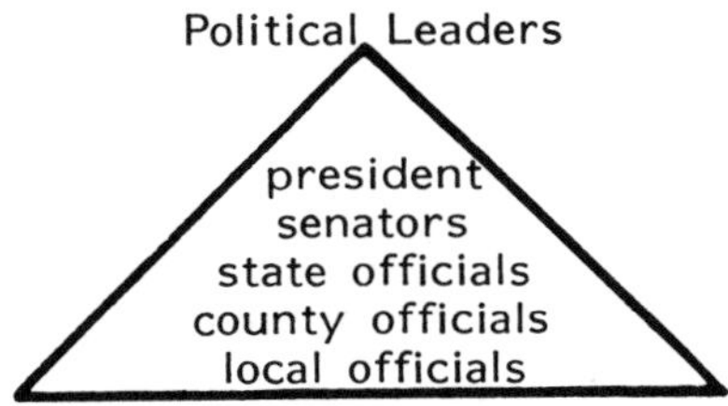


Study the practice fact-bits again. Do you see any other "top to bottom" patterns there? How about:

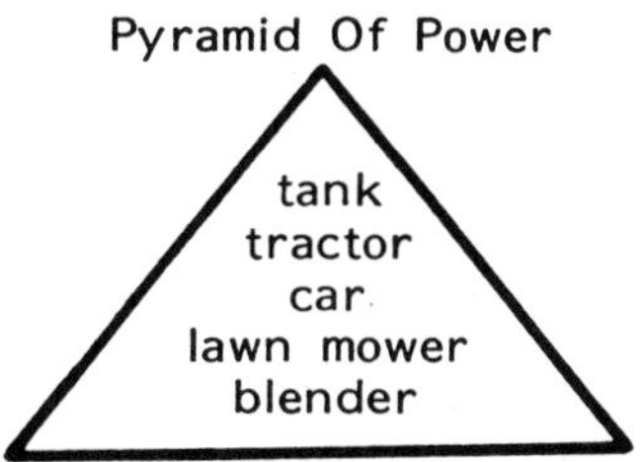


In this Pyramid, you have an arrangement of machines from the most powerful machine at the top to the least powerful at the bottom. Someone else may have seen these machines in a different way and arranged them as follows:

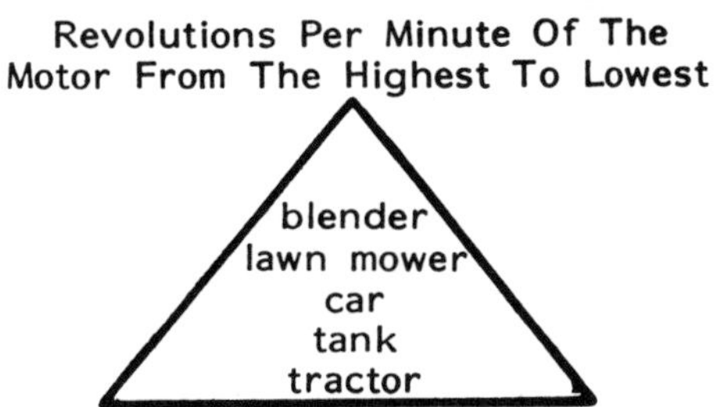


Any number of Pyramids may be found in this list. Here are three more possibilities:

My Favorite
Holidays
Christmas
my birthday
Easter
Things I
Like To Eat
coke
lemons
Things That
Give Off Heat
sun
tank
tractor
car

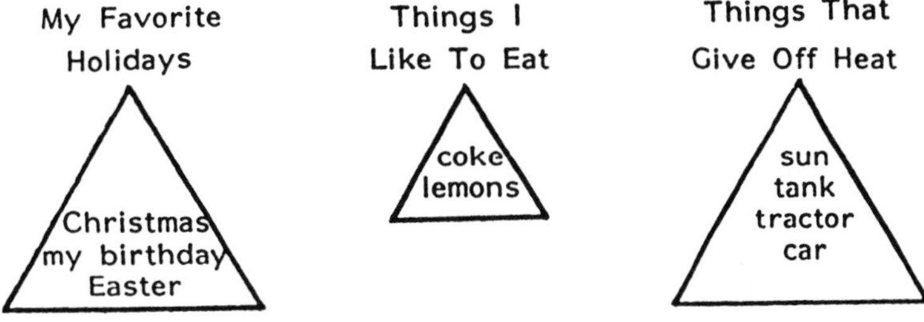

By comparing fact-bits to other fact-bits, you will begin to see relationships that can be put into such a Pyramid. By the way, when finding your own Pyramids, if you think of something that will fit into a Pyramid that you have not included as a fact-bit, feel free to put it into your Pyramid.

It's time to begin doing this on your own. Place your "Smashing: school" page before you again. Take another sheet of paper and refer to your list of fact-bits as you make Pyramids. ATTENTION! FACT-BITS PREVIOUSLY USED IN A *GROUP* MAY BE USED AGAIN IN A PYRAMID. Use fact-bits over and over if you like. Be certain to label each Pyramid, explaining what it contains.

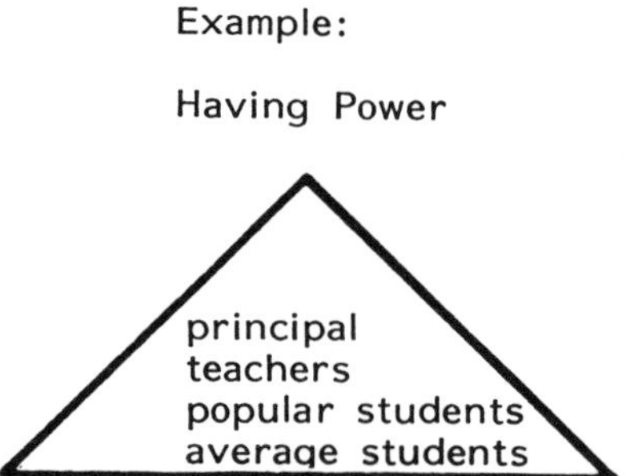


## *Chain*

Now you're ready for the stage of Rearranging called Chain. The Chain is simply another way of shaping the fact-bits on your "Smashing: school" page. A Chain is a sequence of events that does not repeat itself. For instance, if you witnessed a bank robbery, you would explain the event to the police in the following way: "The robbers came into the bank, pulled guns, ordered us to put up our hands, took the money, and ran." This information could be drawn as links of a Chain:

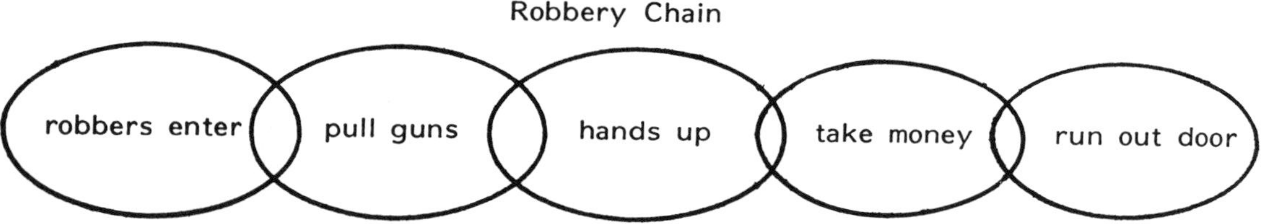


An unfortunate Chain of events might be about children playing with matches:

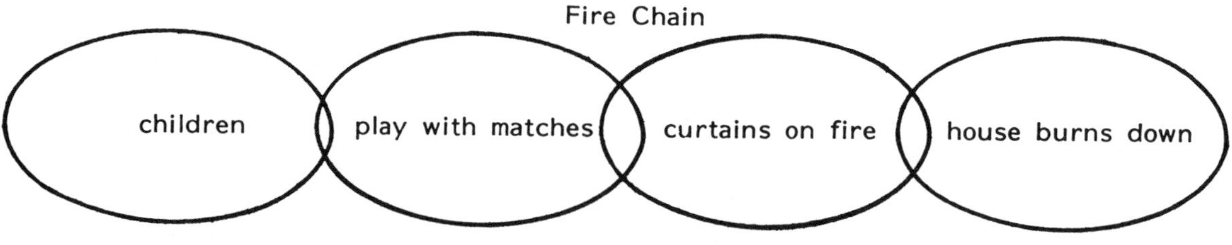

You may also incorporate the same fact-bits you have already used in a Group or Pyramid into a Chain. Do you remember the example of a Pyramid of political leaders?

Political Leaders
president
senators
state officials
county officials
local officials

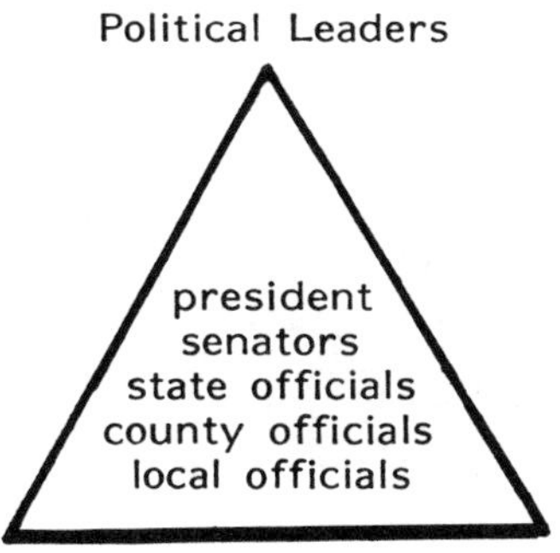

Using the same fact-bits, you could also make the following Chain:

Progress Of A Politician To Greater Power

local official — county official — state official — senator — president

You may think that since you are using the same fact-bits there is no difference between these examples. But there is. "Political leaders" and "progress of a politician to greater power" are entirely different concepts. USE FACT-BITS AGAIN AND AGAIN IF YOU CAN FIT THEM INTO SOME NEW PATTERN.

Take another sheet of paper and make as many Chains from your school fact-bits as you can. Remember, a Chain is a series of fact-bits that does *not* repeat itself. In other words, a Chain is a *one-time* series of events. Draw as many Chains as you can. Work hard at this — it's important. LABEL EACH CHAIN so that you will be able to remember what it represents. You may repeat words you have already used in Groups and Pyramids. Fact-bits may be used again and again!

Example:

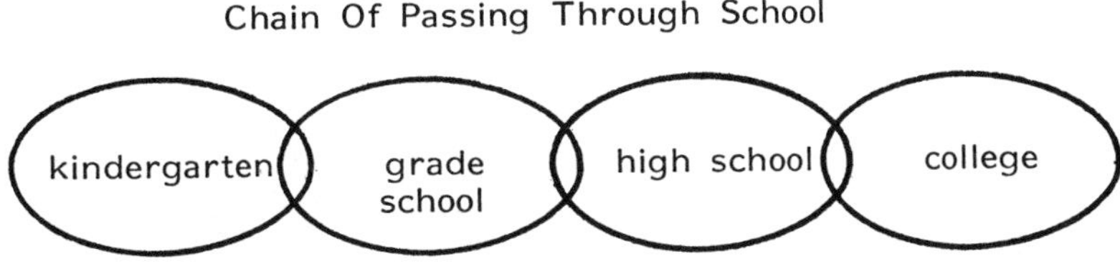

## *Circle*

The fourth and final Rearranging step is the Circle. A Circle is some series of events or incidents that repeats itself. A Circle is a cycle that goes round and round like a dog chasing its tail. Study the three examples of Circles that follow:

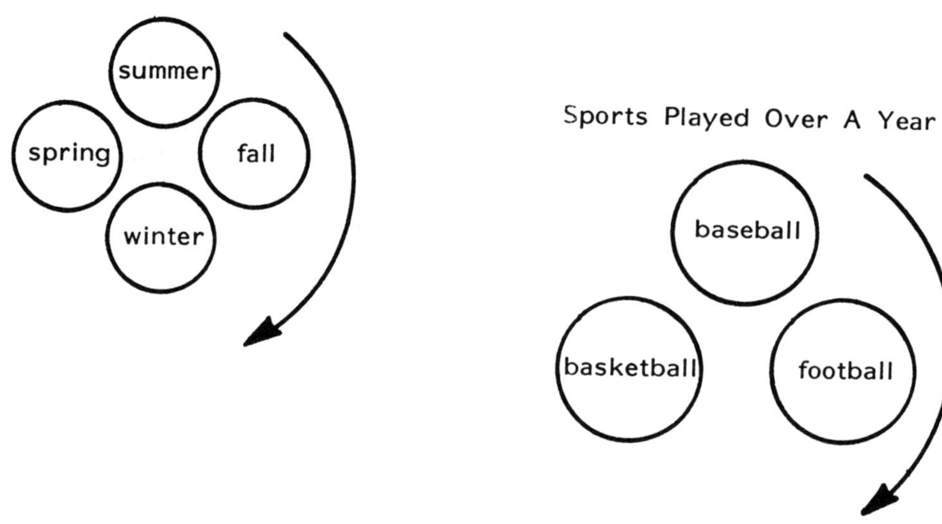


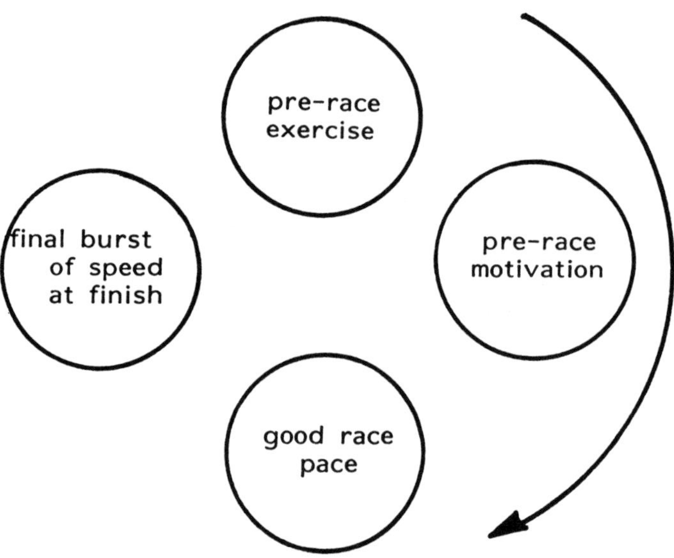


Take a sheet of paper and make as many Circles about school as you can. Include any fact-bits that fit in a Circle, that is, events that go round and round. Be sure to label each Circle so that you will know what it represents later.

Example:

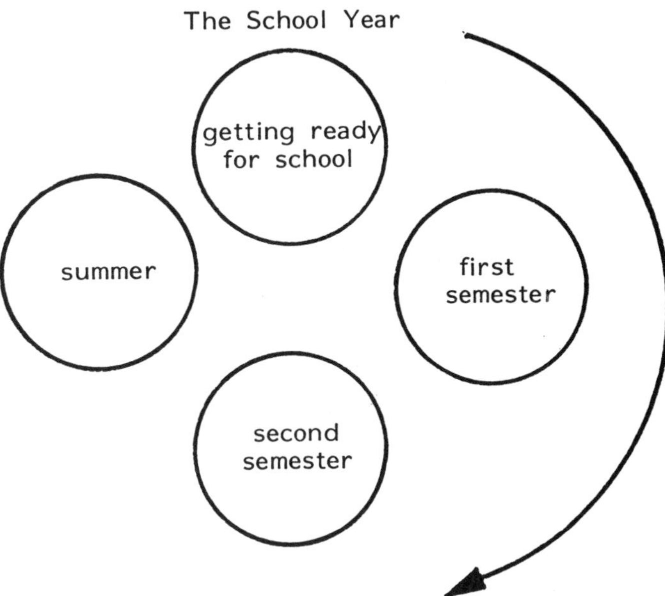


Of the four symbols with which you have been making new organizations of your fact-bits, Circles seem to be the most difficult. Take a little extra time with your Circles. Remember to use old fact-bits if you can.

All you have to do now is make Groups, Pyramids, Chains, and Circles for island. Now that you know what to do, this process will go much faster. Examples, reminding you how to proceed, follow. (If in doubt, turn back to the page explaining the term.) Place your "Smashing: island" page before you, take a blank sheet of paper, and begin.

Make Groups for island. Groups are fact-bits that fit into some category. Here is an example:

Plants

sugar cane
bamboo
grass
oak trees

Be certain to label each Group, showing what you had in mind when you arranged the fact-bits.

Pyramids are items arranged in an order from top to bottom, as in the following example:

Pyramid Of Power

earthquakes
volcanoes
humans plowing
dogs pulling cars

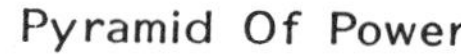

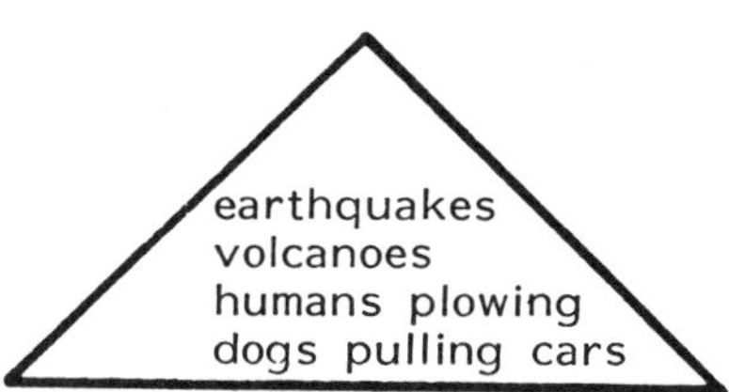

Find Pyramids for island and label them. You may reuse Group fact-bits in your Pyramids. Remember, too, that you may use *any other* fact that fits, even if it is not on your "Smashing: island" page.

A Chain is a sequence of events that does not repeat itself, as this Chain about the growth of a tree illustrates:

Growth Of A Tree

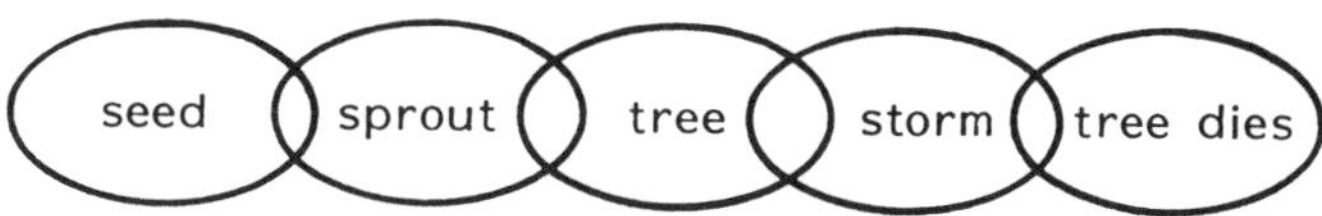


Take a third sheet of paper and make Chains for island; label each one. Fact-bits in Groups and Pyramids may be repeated in Chains. Stray facts may be fitted in, even if they do not appear on your "Smashing: island" page. If a term about island fits into a Chain, put it in.

A Circle is a series of events or incidents that repeats itself.

Circle Of Death

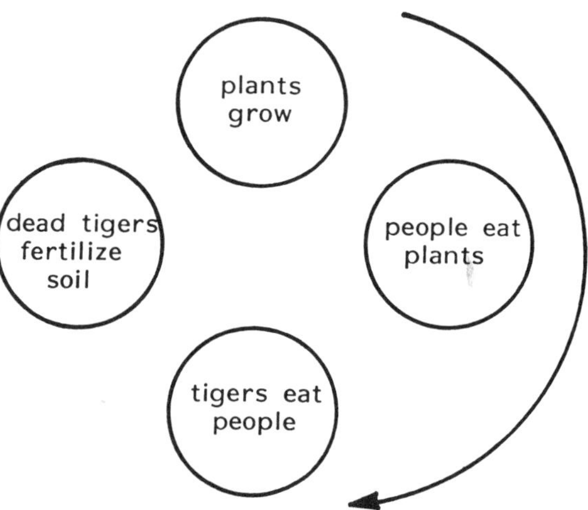


Circles are difficult. On a clean piece of paper make as many Circles about island as you can. Remember, you can use old fact-bits from Groups, Pyramids, and Chains, as well as island fact-bits that have just occurred to you. Label each Circle.

## *Time Out*

What you have just done is make new patterns (Groups, Pyramids, Chains, and Circles) out of your Smashed school and island fact-bits. Since the right brain is the part of your mind that finds new patterns from old information, this process called on you to use your inventive right brain. But that's not all you did. You also labeled or titled each new pattern, indicating what it (whether Group, Pyramid, Chain, or Circle) contained. If you have not done this, GO BACK IMMEDIATELY AND DO IT NOW!

By the way, did you have some trouble thinking of a label for some categories? Most people do. But why? If you know enough to put fact-bits into some sort of organization, you should have no difficulty finding a *heading*. But that is not always the case. Making *patterns* is a creative, *right-brain* function. Saying a *name* (language) is a *left-brain* function. In effect, you have to shift back and forth, using both halves of your brain to do your Rearranging — not an easy thing to do. This shifting, or switching, is much like the experience most of us have had of recognizing someone (a right-brain function), but not being able to say the person's *name* (a left-brain function), or feeling on the verge of making an important discovery, but having trouble *saying* what it is.

**Stop!**

You are much too tired to continue. In fact, this is all you should do on this problem for the rest of the day. Put this book away. Rest tonight; start again tomorrow.

Now that your brain is rested, you may begin again: let's hope this time off has served as an Incubation period.

You have already had the chance to think up some similarities between school and island by fact-bit comparison in Creating I (page 56). Now look for more similarities between school and island in Creating II.

## *Creating II*

First, study the four pages of Groups, Pyramids, Chains, and Circles for school and the four similar pages for island. Stack the two piles of pages before you, with the Group pages on top. Next, look at your drawings of school and island again, checking to see if there is something else in your pictures you would like to include in a Group. Then put away the picture page and concentrate on your Group fact-bits, refreshing your memory by rereading them several times.

You're now almost ready to begin the last stage of LARC III, Creating II, in which you compare your Groups, Pyramids, Chains, and Circles for *school* to the same patterns you made for *island*. These patterns, made from your Smashed fact-bits, should help you see similarities between school and island. Record any creative ideas you get from this process on your "Similarities between school and island" answer sheet.

But first, to give you an idea how this is done, let's take several examples from a different problem, one finding similarities between "society" and the "body." The following two Groups have been created under these categories:

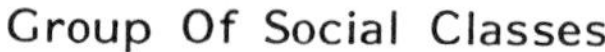


upper class
middle class
lower class

Ruled By The Brain

legs, arms
emotions
impulses

By comparing these Groups, someone discovered the following similarity:

> Both show that a ruling part makes decisions for the rest. In social classes, this is the upper class; in the case of the body, it is the brain.

Can you see that this similarity was discovered when the subject saw "upper class" at the top of the "Social Classes" Group, then noticed that the "brain" was controlling "legs," "emotions," and "impulses"? In this case, the similarity was between "upper class ruling" and "brain ruling."

In another example, a subject compared a Group from society with a Chain from body.

Society Is Organized

social classes
laws

Chain Of Body Functioning

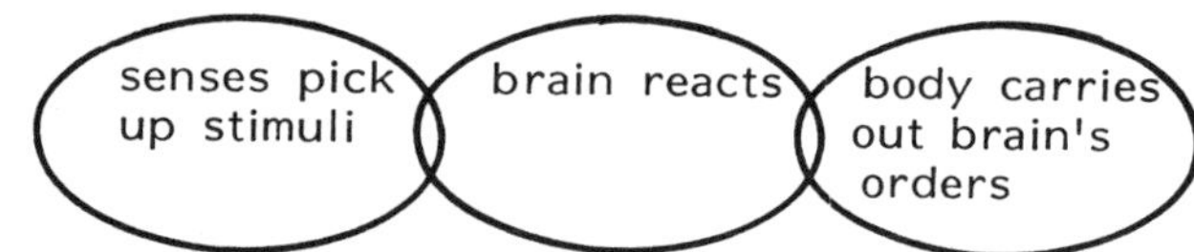


The subject came up with this simple similarity:

> Society has different parts. These are the various social classes. The body has different parts—the senses, the brain, and the body parts that do what the brain says.

A more complex similarity was given:

> Both society and the brain function best when they are organized. Laws make a society run smoothly, and the body runs best when the brain is in control.

This idea was generated comparing this Group to this Chain. (Note: when you reach this stage, you will be comparing not only Groups to Groups, Pyramids to Pyramids, etc., but also Groups to Pyramids, Pyramids to Circles, and so on.)

This is difficult! Let's take a few more examples so it will be clear to you what the possibilities are before you compare your Groups, Pyramids, Chains, and Circles about school and island. In the society-body comparison, the following Group was matched against a Pyramid:

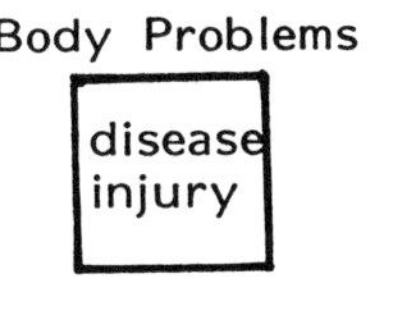


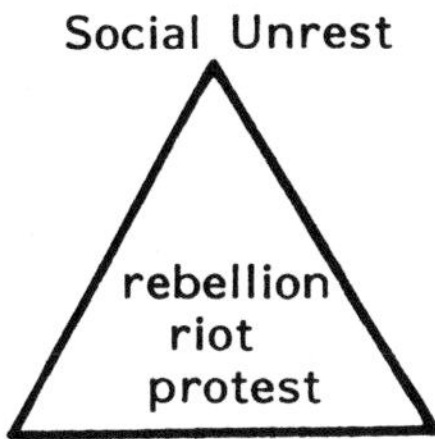


The subject came up with a rather complex similarity: both have "types of disruption."

In the final sample problem — how is "baseball" like "studying" — the following Groups were compared:

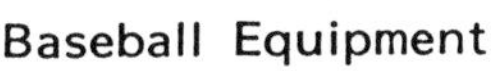


bats
uniforms
lights
players

Studying Equipment

books
pens
study lamps
students

Some connections are (1) they both have lights — night baseball and the study lamps; (2) they both have people — baseball players and students; (3) they both require physical objects — bats for baseball, pens for students.

Now see what similarities you can find between island and school. Compare the titles of your Groups for school to titles of your Groups for island. Do you see any similarities between school and island? What about the words inside the Groups? What similarities do you find? Next, compare your island Groups to your school Pyramids. Then compare island Groups to school Chains. Continue this process until you have exhausted all possibilities.

This final step is the most important because you are ACTUALLY CREATING. Find as many similarities between school and island as you can. Write each one on the "similarities between school and island" page. Some similarities, having nothing to do with any pattern or fact-bits, may come to you "out of the blue." Write those down also. Go ahead. Create!

It's time now to turn back to the original list of similarities between school and island that you made early in the chapter (page 52). (This was the one you did before using LARC.) Compare the similarities you just discovered using LARC for school and island to the similarities you got on your own. You should find not only that LARC has helped you to see many more similarities, but also that several of them are more . . . interesting. While many people increase both the number and the complexity of their list of similarities the first time they use LARC, others need a couple of run-throughs with LARC before making similar progress. Interestingly, the speed with which a person learns LARC has little to do with the amount or quality of creativity that person eventually achieves. After all, practice affects most activities — from riding a bicycle to becoming more creative. The learning style of some people simply takes longer than that of others. But, as in most things, it is the end product that counts.

## How Others Did

Before closing this chapter, let's discuss the lists of similarities produced by some of the subjects who helped in the process of testing LARC. In general, these people wrote down three types of similarities for school and island, the first of which we call "playful." One person said that birds flying over school or island would leave their droppings on each. Another wrote that you could make a liverwurst sandwich in a school and on an island. Though these answers are certainly creative, you might ask, "Do such answers have any value?" While they may be of no use to you, they might be just what a *comedian* needs, comedy often relying on surprise and strangeness for its effect. What might be a wasted response to one person might not be for another.

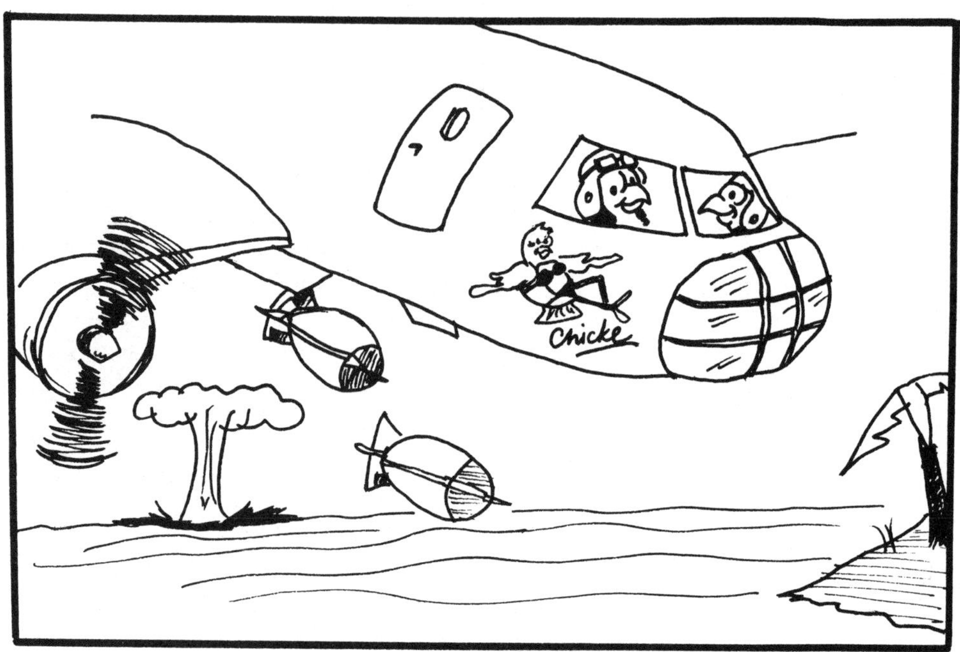


A second category of answers was what can be called "simple." Subjects did a lot of matching grass on the island with grass in the school yard, sand with sand, trees with trees, people with people.

The third category of similarities may be called "complex" or "higher-level" responses. It's interesting to examine some of these answers. One subject, for instance, compared the following school Group to island Pyramid:

Things Learned In School

knowledge of subjects
how to date
how to be social
skills--typing
physical education

Island Pyramid Of Beauty

nature
sunset
beach

About this comparison the subject wrote:

> Both school and island have romance. You learn about romantic stories at school, in *Romeo and Juliet,* and you make dates there. On an island you have a romantic setting.

Notice that the word "romance" didn't appear in either the school Group or the island Pyramid. But by looking at the list in each, you can probably see how the subject came up with romance as something similar between school and island.

Let's take another example of what seems to be higher creativity as generated by LARC. The subject produced the following Chain and Circle:

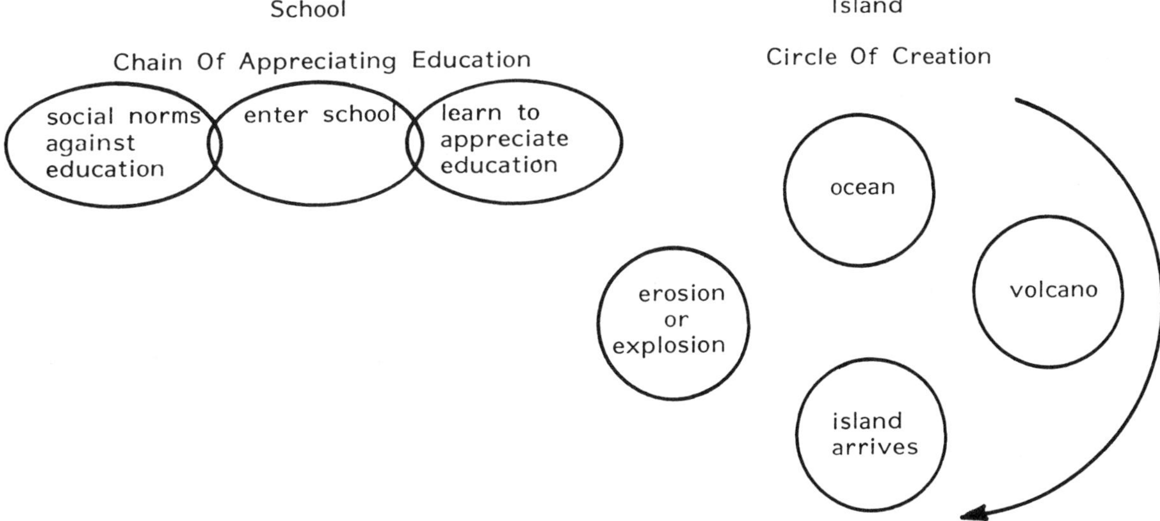


When comparing this Chain to this Circle, the subject discovered:

> Both school and island have boundaries that separate them from the mass: in the case of an island, the mass is the ocean; in the case of the school, it is society.

A final example illustrates how even the most complex ideas coming from a direct comparison of fact-bits (Creating I) do not always require the use of organizing tools. The subject giving this response noted that the idea "came to him" when he compared the fact-bit "develops one's view of life" (from school — "characteristics") with "thick jungle — clear horizon" (from island — "sight images of").

> Both school and island have clear and cloudy vision: in the case of island, if you look inland toward the jungle, you can't see much and what you do see would be distorted by shadows and the jungle. In the case of school, when you arrive, you have a cloudy vision as represented by fuzzy concepts. On an island, your vision would be clear as you turn to look over the ocean, just as in a school, as you are educated you learn to see things clearly.

## Review

Throughout the problem, you were given tasks to perform, some of them designed to force the right (creative) side of your brain to work, others designed to force the left (logical) side of your brain to function. For to be creative, information must switch back and forth between the halves of the brain. The entire brain must get into the inventive act.

In addition, most of you have seen that LARC works, even with a hypothetical problem (school-island similarity). With a problem of real interest, LARC will work even better, particularly as you practice and begin putting into operation suggestions presented later in the book. (But for now, it is time – before you forget it – to THROW AWAY YOUR PICTURES OF SCHOOL AND ISLAND BEFORE SOMEONE SEES THEM!)

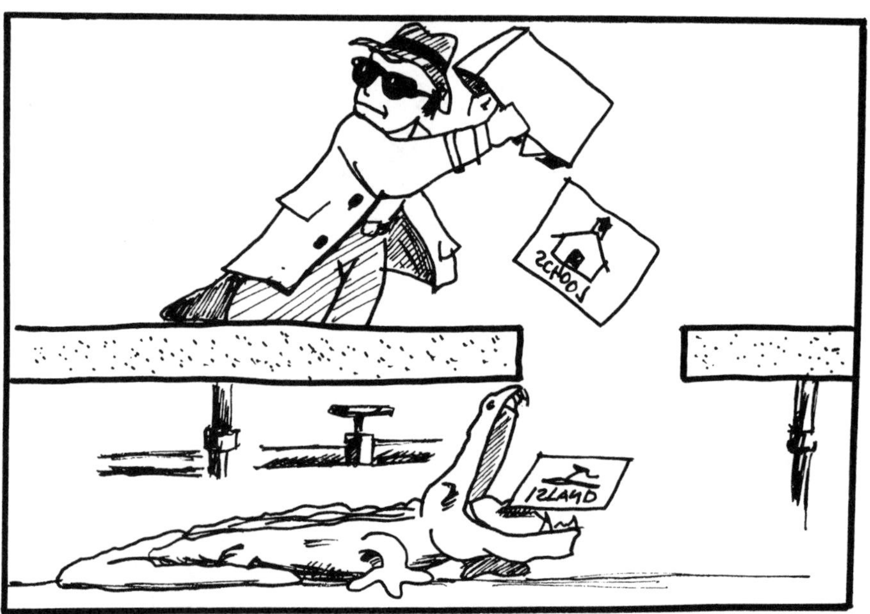


## Just for Fun

After all this work, you deserve a story. So sit back, relax, enjoy.

The hero of the tale is that great ancient Greek philosopher, Thales; the subject, "natural creativity" and its relation to LARC.

### Thales' Day in the Sun

Once upon a time, Thales of Miletus (640?–546 B.C.) was given the task of measuring the height of the Great Pyramid in Egypt – no mean feat for two reasons: (1) the Great Pyramid is four hundred and eighty-one feet tall (as tall as a thirty-story office building), and (2) as a pyramid, its sides slope from apex to base. Measuring a side would give a figure *greater* than the pyramid's height. It's a nasty little problem, no doubt of that!

Had he been alive today, Thales would, quite naturally, have rushed right out to buy a copy of this book as an aid to this puzzle's solution – *so-o-o* – let's imagine what would have happened if he had used LARC III on this tricky problem of pyramid measurement.

First, since the two key words in the problem before him (measuring the height of the Great Pyramid of Giza) are "pyramid" and "measure," Thales would have chosen to process them through LARC. He would start – do you believe it? – by drawing pictures of a pyramid (or pyramids), then of some methods of measure:

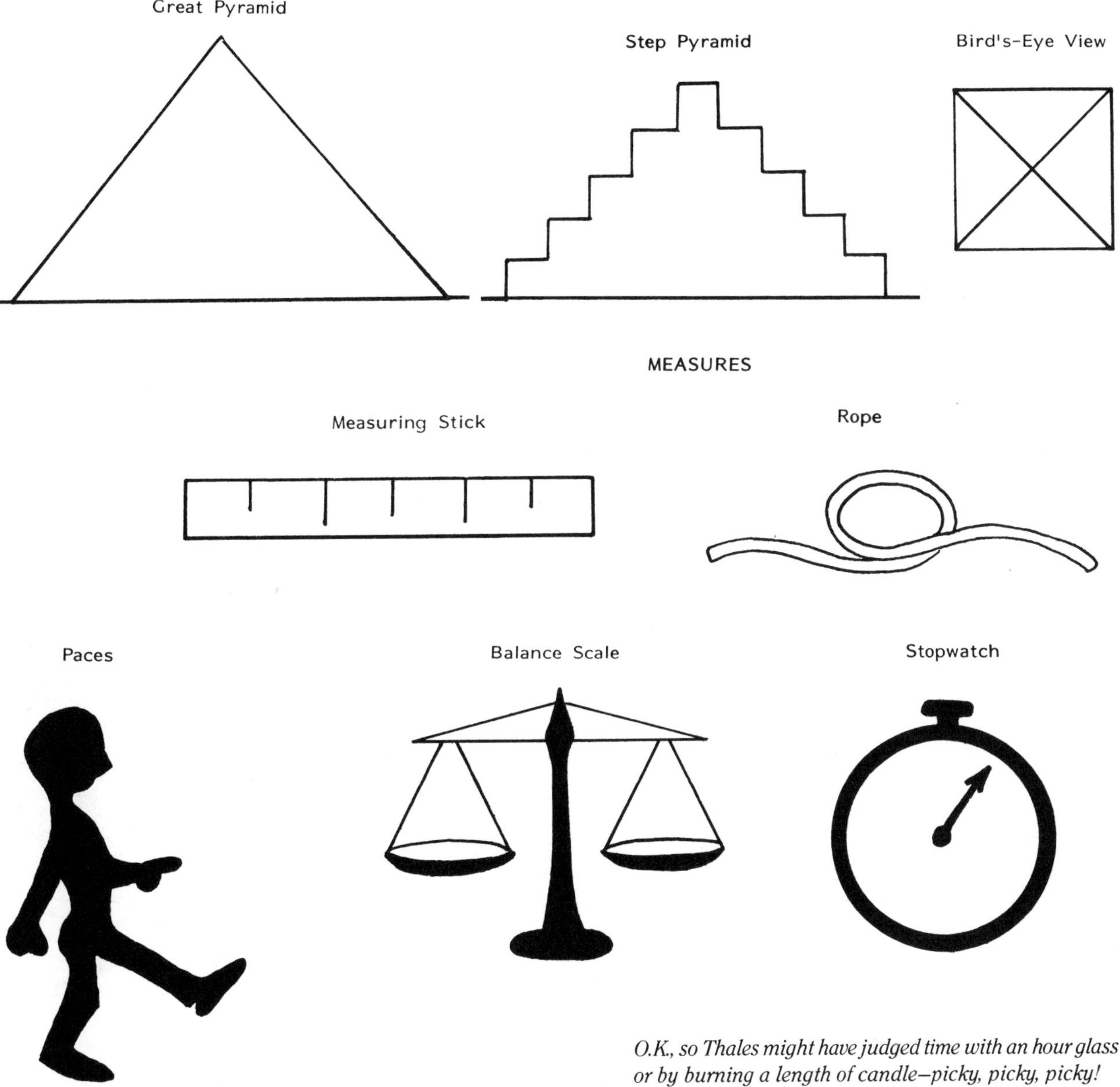


*O.K., so Thales might have judged time with an hour glass or by burning a length of candle–picky, picky, picky!*

Thales would then have smashed his drawings into fact-bits.

### *Smashing: pyramid*

3. Parts — *stones, height*
12. Things connected with — *sky, background, sand at base, sun overhead, shadow on sand; everything on earth is of same elements; I am to pyramid as an ant in desert is to me*
17. Touching images of — *it's hot standing in sun looking up at it, cooler in pyramid's shadow*
18. Characteristics — *sloping sides; looks different at night — shadows; too tall to build ladder to measure; looks bigger close up; shadow longer in morning and evening*

### *Smashing: measures*

1. Types — *yardstick, pace off, time, rope*
18. Characteristics — *length of slant*

We'll skip Creating I for now and look at how Thales would have handled Rearranging. He would place his fact-bits inside organizing symbols: Groups, Pyramids, Chains, and Circles.

Pyramid

All Parts

stone
sand
horizon
shadow

Chain Up

foundation
stone
sky

Day In Life Of Pyramid

sunrise, one side bright, shadow long

noon--no shadow, all sides lit

evening, other side bright, shadow long

night--dark dark as I walk around the giant

Life And Death Circle

rocks built into pyramid

sand of desert blows--erodes

eons change pyramid dust to rock again

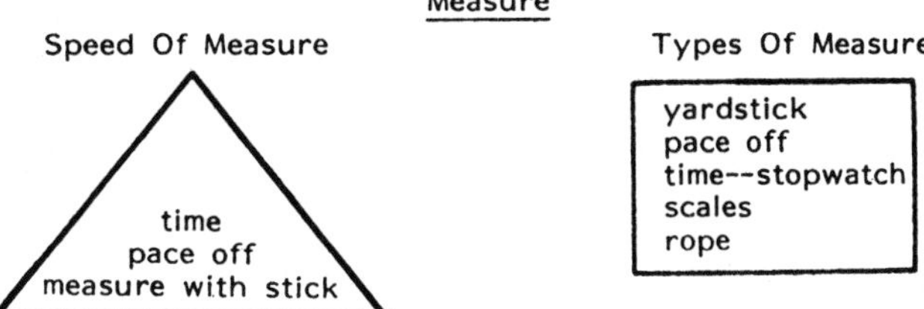


In Creating I and Creating II, Thales would have the following thoughts about a possible solution:

1. Pace off; walk up side; won't work.
2. Use rope to measure — hang down from point. No good; would get measurement of the side — the slope, not the height.
3. Use time as a measure. Drop a rock; time drop with stopwatch, knowing how fast it would accelerate. No, would hit side of slope, not the ground.
4. Drill a hole through the pyramid from top to bottom, drop rope in hole. No, stone too hard, and Pharaoh would kill me for defacing his pyramid.
5. If this were just the step pyramid, could measure the steps, then add them.

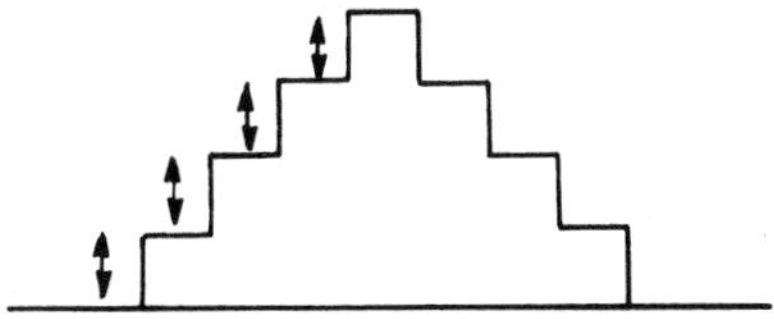

Could get the same result by gouging holes in sides of pyramid. No, Pharaoh would kill me for defacing pyramid.

6. Could shoot a straight flying bird just as it took off from the top of the pyramid, waiting until it had cleared the base so that it would fall straight down on the sand, then time the bird's fall . . .

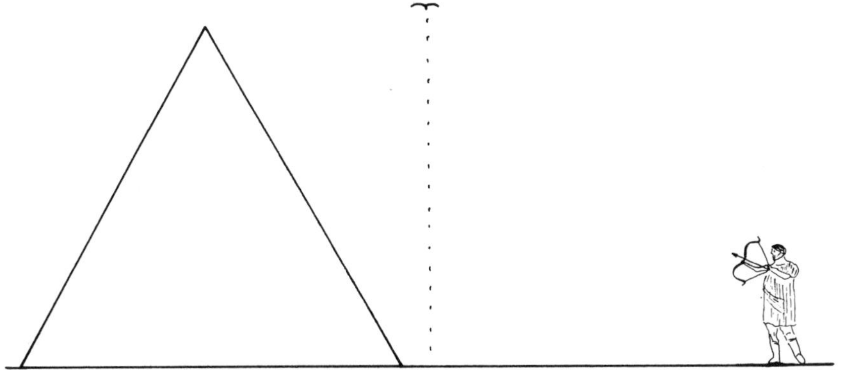

I must be getting a fever from standing out in the hot sun too long!

7. Put a board across the apex, then measure straight down. Impractical.

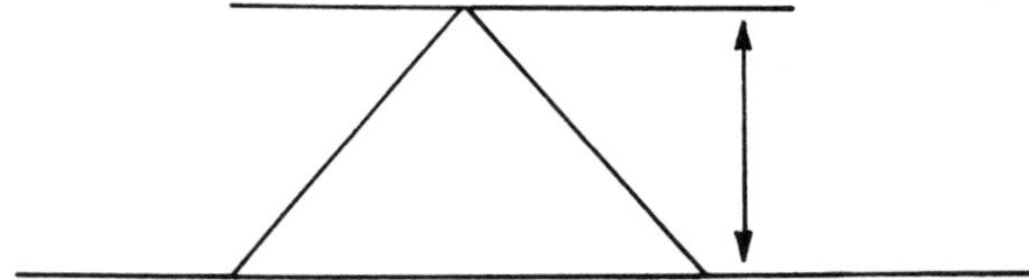

8. Wait for the pyramid to erode, until it's my size, then eye-ball across the top. . . . No doubt about it, I'm not a well man!
9. I need to change something so that I can measure it. But what can change? It looks darker at night and lighter in the daytime. Hmm. The shadow length also changes. The length of time I've been standing here has put me in the shade, thank the gods, since the pyramid's shadow has lengthened this afternoon. An ant beside me would also be grateful for being in *my* shadow on a hot day like this. THAT'S IT!

What has he found? Think about it, then read on for Thales' solution.

Though everything casts a shadow in relation to its own height (*tall* things cast *long* shadows, *short* things cast *short* shadows),Thales noticed that shadow lengths change throughout the day — both the shadow length of the pyramid and his own shadow length. As the sun swings overhead (Thales wouldn't have known about the earth's rotation) an object's shadow will lengthen or shorten depending on the angle of the sun to that object. The solution Thales was seeking? Thales first measured his own height, then stood in the desert beside the pyramid. He watched until his own shadow grew to be exactly the same length as his real height. Reasoning that, at that moment, the pyramid's shadow would also equal its height, Thales measured the structure's shadow to get the correct answer.

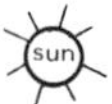


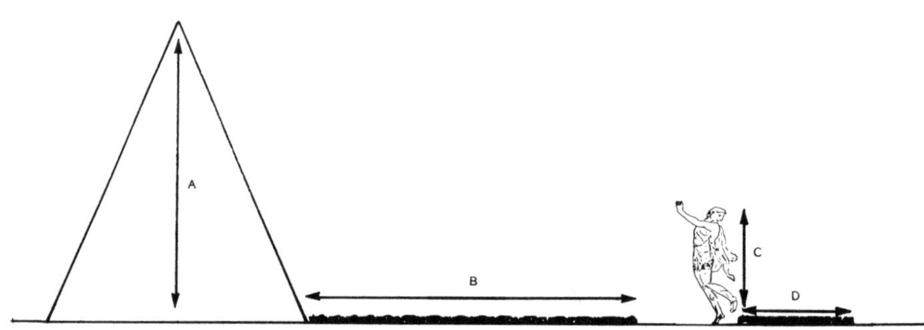


*Line A is the same length as line B.*
*Line C is the same length as line D.*

Of course, we've just been pretending that Thales used LARC (though you may be sure that, if it had been available to him, he *would* have used it — ahem), but we can speculate that his thought processes were something like those LARC *causes.* For highly creative people, right-left brain shifts are so rapid, so subtle, even *they* don't recognize what's happening when they have an idea "pop" into their minds.

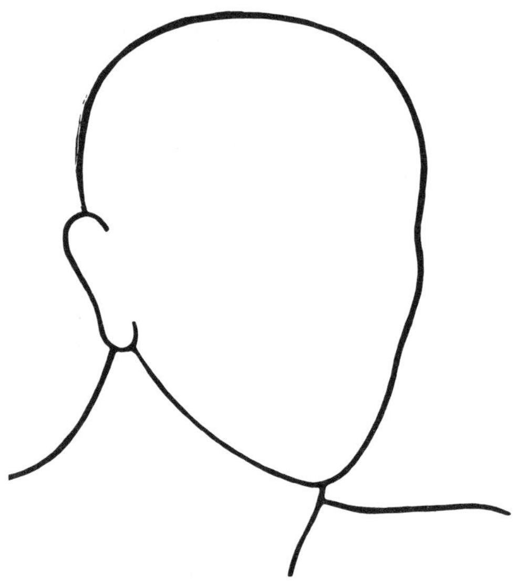

# 6
# LARC IV: The Works

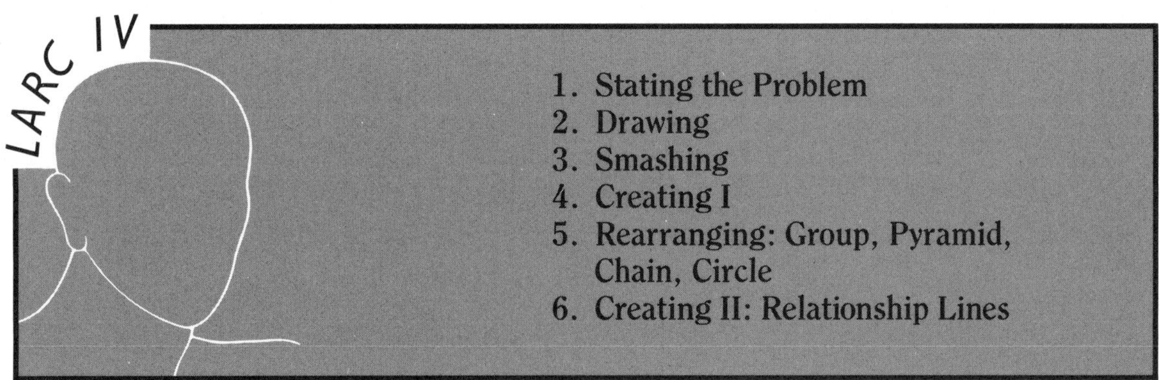


So far, two problems have been run through LARC, an easy problem (finding uses for a brick) and a harder problem ("school and island" similarity). The key to each solution has been "breaking down" essential terms or patterns (brick, school, island). A question that has not been addressed, however, is just what terms to break down (smash). And that is the first topic, as we pursue *LARC IV: The Works*.

## *Stating the Problem*

When working problems of your own, you may encounter difficulty deciding just what terms need to be smashed. Helping you arrive at this decision is the purpose of "Stating the Problem," a step that you may want to add to simpler versions of LARC. When Stating the Problem, write the problem on a piece of paper several times, varying your sentences. Try to make your thoughts more *specific*. If you pursue the term "game," for instance, when what you really want to know about is "football," the more general term will produce responses about badminton, polo, hockey—all of which are irrelevant to what you really want: information about *football.* Or, you may attempt to pursue what will make you "happy," when what you need are ideas about how to be *happy* on a limited supply of *money*.

Let's take a detailed example. Suppose you are a publicist making a sports film. You could run "sports" and "film" through LARC – but before you do, you should explore the problem carefully to see if other terms might be more specific, more apt to yield valuable ideas. To do this, ask yourself what kind of sports film. You might write another sentence: I want to make a sports film about football. Then you would think about what you want to include in such a film – excitement, something about the team, information to help the school recruit athletes for the program, etc. Finally, you write: I want to make a highlight film on my college football program that will be exciting and also informative and inspirational to potential recruits. (This is really what you wanted to do all along; it just took a few sentences to explain it to yourself.)

Next, you must decide what parts (key terms) of your problem you want to run through LARC. Looking at the final sentence about the sports film, you notice the word "football" as well as "film" is important. Anything else? Hmm. This is certainly a more difficult problem than finding uses for a brick. The "brick" problem was "simple," in part because it wasn't very important. This highlight film is more complex than the "school and island" similarity search, and – how could it be otherwise? – more valuable. Because this problem could really make a difference between a good or poor film, it might make sense to trace *more* than two concepts through LARC. How about, in addition to football and film, smashing the words "excitement" and "recruits"?

After Stating the Problem and choosing the key terms, the next step is drawing.

## Drawing

Draw. . . . What? Let's continue with the film example. For film, you could sketch a picture of a camera, perhaps, or of a piece of film, or produce a picture of you shooting the film. For college football, you might show someone catching a pass, or a stadium, or goalposts – whatever college football means to *you*, however you see it in *your* mind. For recruits, you might sketch men in letter sweaters. But for excitement? At this point, you have to make a symbolic drawing, perhaps something completely unrelated to football or film. If you find exploring Africa the most exciting thing you can imagine, then a map of Africa is what you need at this point. If your mind turns to college girls as cheerleaders, then you should draw them doing cheers. Draw whatever you think is exciting; this will stimulate your right brain.

Another point to make about the Drawing stage is that the more detail you can put into your pictures, the better. Make pictures from several perspectives, as you did when drawing your brick. For the maximum effort, find an actual object, an object that means (to you) something about one of your pictures, and bring it to your desk. You might get your movie camera and put it beside you, picking it up to look at it as you proceed with LARC. Although it's not mandatory, having an object can't hurt. The creative right brain is pictorial; give it what it wants – two-dimensional images, three-dimensional objects.

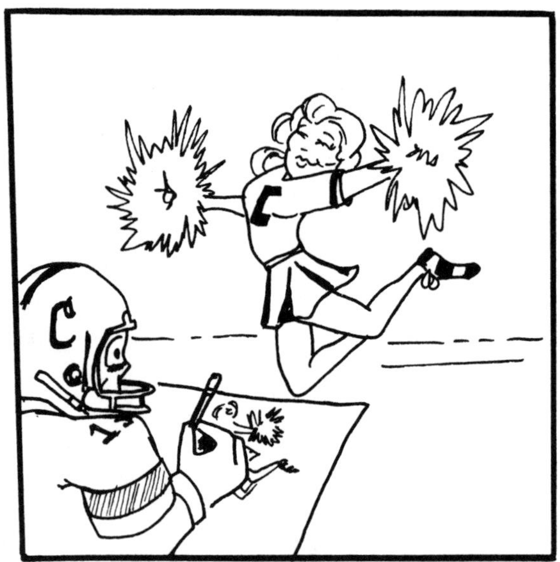

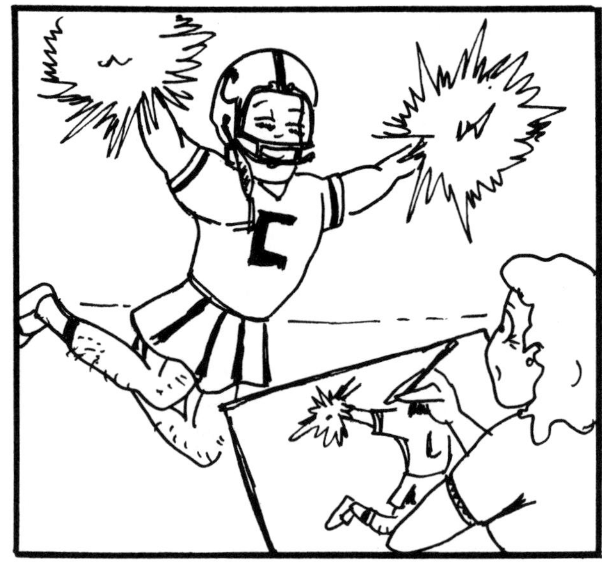

## *Smashing*

You have been given four sets of Smashing words and phrases from which to choose, depending on the nature of the problem you are trying to solve. The lists are as follows:

*Passive*

| *Simple* | *Complex* |
|---|---|
| 1. Types | 1. Types |
| 2. Steps | 2. Steps |
| 3. Parts | 3. Parts |
| 4. Causes | 4. Causes |
| 5. When | 5. Synonyms |
| 6. Why | 6. Who |
| 7. How | 7. What |
| 8. Things connected with | 8. When |
| 9. Sight images of | 9. Where |
| 10. Products or results | 10. Why |
| | 11. How |
| | 12. Things connected with |
| | 13. Sight images of |
| | 14. Hearing images of |
| | 15. Emotions |
| | 16. Opposite |
| | 17. Touching images of |
| | 18. Characteristics |
| | 19. Products or results |
| | 20. Modes of operation |

*Active*

| *Simple* | *Complex* |
|---|---|
| 1. Abilities | 1. Abilities |
| 2. Fear or threats | 2. Fear or threats |
| 3. Goals and hopes | 3. Goals and hopes |
| 4. Strengths | 4. Responsibilities |
| 5. Weaknesses | 5. Interests |
| 6. Types | 6. Likes |
| 7. Steps | 7. Dislikes |
| 8. Things connected with | 8. Strengths |
| 9. Sight images of | 9. Weaknesses |
| 10. Characteristics | 10. Types |
| | 11. Causes |
| | 12. Steps |
| | 13. How become |
| | 14. Who is |
| | 15. Where |
| | 16. When |
| | 17. Things connected with |
| | 18. Sight images of |
| | 19. Characteristics |
| | 20. Products or results |

Choose the list that seems most appropriate for the problem with which you are working and begin smashing your terms.

## Breakthroughs

One other bit of advice (which applies throughout LARC) is LOOK OUT FOR BREAKTHROUGHS! A breakthrough is a sudden idea, even the very solution for which you have been looking, which can come to you at any time. You're doing your drawings or your smashing when, suddenly, you get an idea. This happened to some of our subjects on the "school and island" problem. And they *complained* about it! "We keep getting these ideas and it's not yet *time* for ideas." It was as if they were being disloyal to LARC by being creative *too soon*. *Now hear this*! It is *never* too soon to have a creative idea! Not having any sense of timing, your right brain may give you a breakthrough at any time of the day or night. Accept such inspiration gratefully, hurrying to write down your idea before you forget it.

## Creating I

Record all answers gotten by fact-bit comparison on your answer sheet.

## *Rearranging*

Make Groups, Pyramids, Chains, and Circles from your fact-bits. After doing that, draw a small picture beside each of these organizing symbols, a picture representing what the symbol means to you. This is another way to trigger the pictorial nature of your right brain. For instance, if you have a Group labeled "Destruction," you might make a line drawing of a mushroom-shaped cloud beside it, a plate breaking, or a firecracker going off — anything that *means* destruction to *you*.

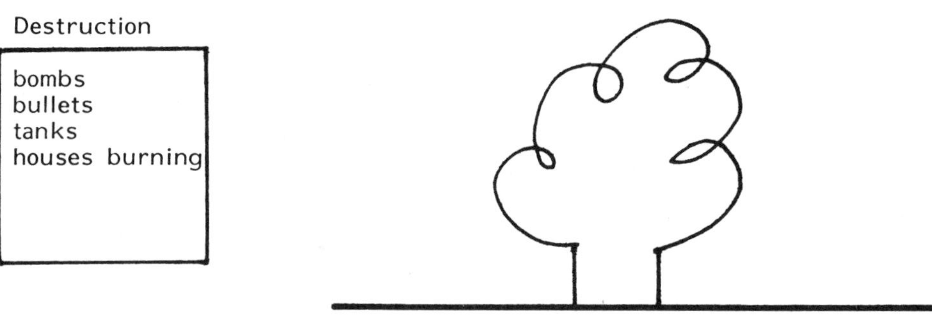


In like manner, you might draw a miniature factory beside a Pyramid labeled "factory."

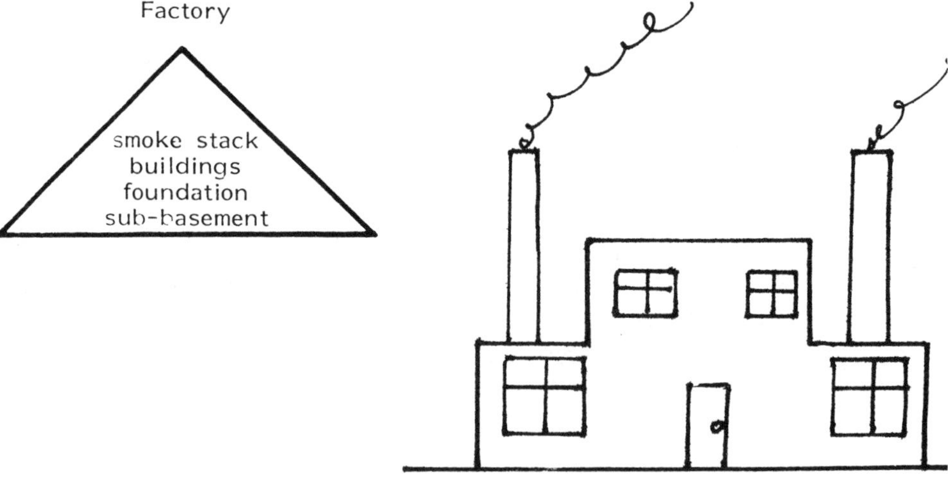


A single fact-bit may seem so important that you want to consider it all by itself. If that happens, just put a box around that single fact-bit. Give it a title, if you like.

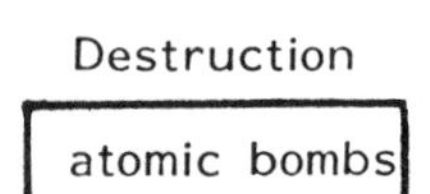

You may, when looking at a number of organizing symbols, regroup their titles under an additional symbol. For instance:

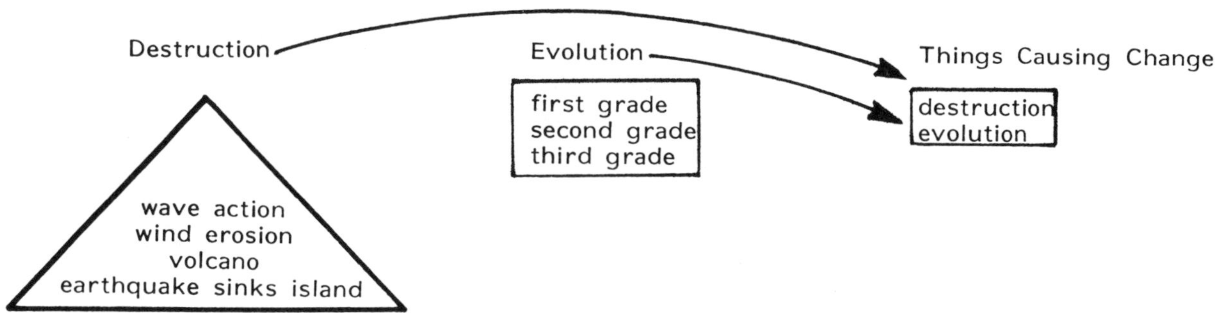


## *Creating II*

As with LARC II and III, the final step of LARC IV is Creating II. But before you proceed to a comparison of organizing symbols (Groups, Pyramids, etc.), try drawing what we call "Relationship Lines" to connect those symbols you feel might be matched with each other in some way. For instance, as in the following symbols, you may draw a line to emphasize an interesting relationship:

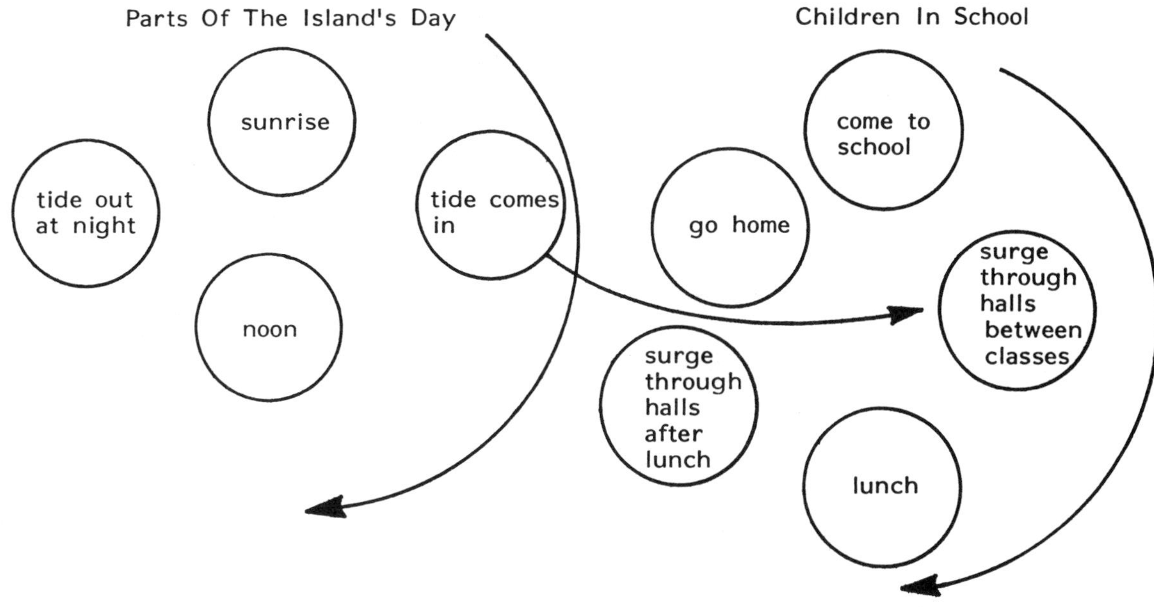


Drawing this connecting line may make it easier for you to see the following similarity: as the tide comes in regularly on the island, so do the children flood the school's halls at regular intervals between their classes.

You may want to draw any or all of the following four lines, each to represent some comparing or contrasting relationship between the organizing symbols.

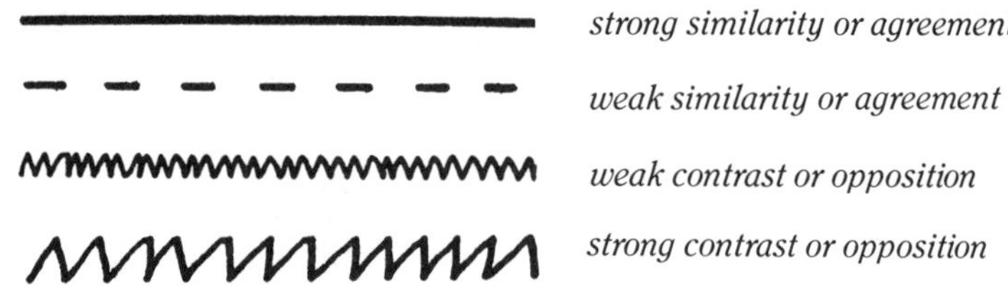


Another example of how these lines might be valuable could be for a college president faced with the question: how can I best spend my limited budget at the college? Everyone on the faculty wants money spent on his or her department, of course, so this hypothetical president runs "college" through LARC. Finally, the president comes up with the following Groups:

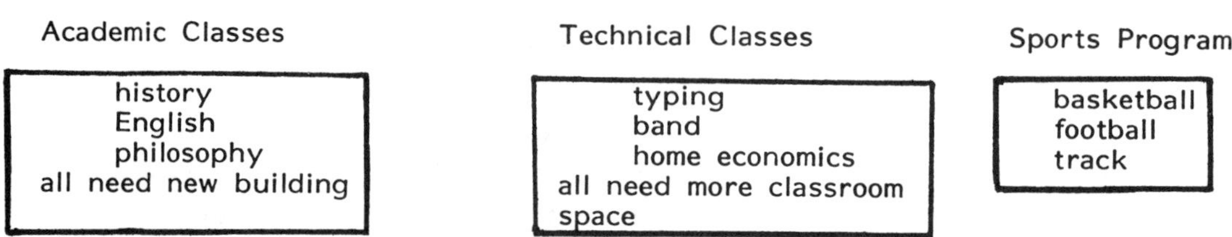


Our president begins to draw Relationship Lines as an aid to clear thinking about the budget.

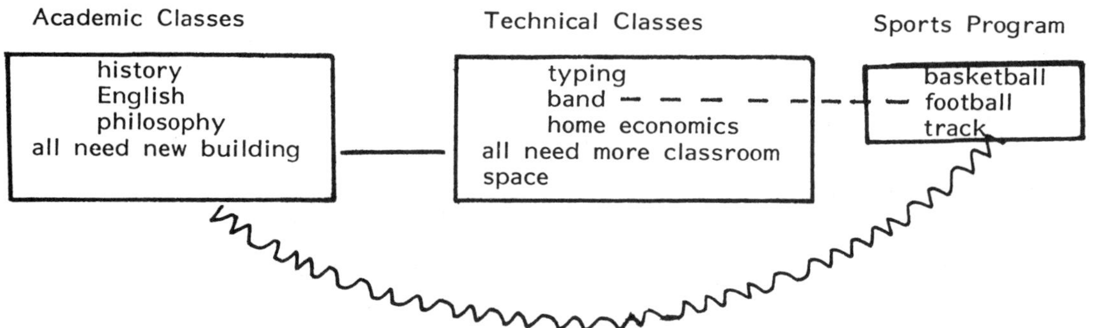


Some of these lines indicate that there is a conflict between spending money on academic classes and spending the same money on the sports program. Since the band marches at halftime, spending money on the band might help the football program. But the strong agreement line is between the need of academic classes for a new building and the need of the technical classes for more classroom space. Perhaps spending money on a new building that both groups could use would satisfy two objectives. That might be the solution.

If you're not generating many creative responses, here is a final suggestion. Put each of your Groups, Pyramids, Chains, and Circles on a 3″ x 5″ card. It's easy to shuffle the cards and match the symbols against each other.

And that's it. You now understand LARC IV.

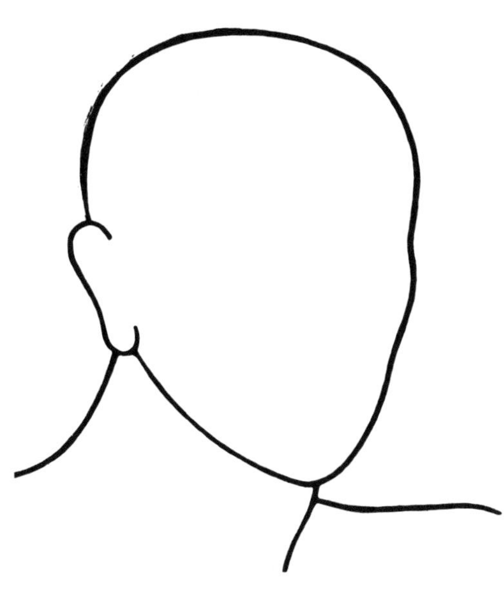

# 7 LARC: In Brief

In the course of the book, four versions of LARC have been presented, each progressively more detailed, the simpler versions, LARC I and LARC II, to be tried first, the more complex, LARC III and IV, for difficult or "stubborn" problems. Now that you have learned the basics of LARC, you need checklists (uncluttered by unnecessary instructions) to help you with problems of your own. Four checklists for LARC I through IV follow.

## LARC I

1. **Drawing:** Draw pictures of each word or concept you will use in the program.
   A. Draw specific pictures for specific terms (house, school) and symbolic pictures for symbolic terms (destruction, love).
   B. Draw several pictures from different angles, perspectives, etc., for each word.
2. **Smashing:** Use one of the four following lists — active, passive, simple, complex — to generate fact-bits from your terms.

*Passive*

| *Simple* | *Complex* |
|---|---|
| 1. Types | 1. Types |
| 2. Steps | 2. Steps |
| 3. Parts | 3. Parts |
| 4. Causes | 4. Causes |
| 5. When | 5. Synonyms |
| 6. Why | 6. Who |
| 7. How | 7. What |
| 8. Things connected with | 8. When |
| 9. Sight images of | 9. Where |
| 10. Products or results | 10. Why |

*(continued)*

*Complex*

11. How
12. Things connected with
13. Sight images of
14. Hearing images of
15. Emotions
16. Opposite
17. Touching images of
18. Characteristics
19. Products or results
20. Modes of operation

*Active*

*Simple*

1. Abilities
2. Fear or threats
3. Goals and hopes
4. Strengths
5. Weaknesses
6. Types
7. Steps
8. Things connected with
9. Sight images of
10. Characteristics

*Complex*

1. Abilities
2. Fear or threats
3. Goals and hopes
4. Responsibilities
5. Interests
6. Likes
7. Dislikes
8. Strengths
9. Weaknesses
10. Types
11. Causes
12. Steps
13. How become
14. Who is
15. Where
16. When
17. Things connected with
18. Sight images of
19. Characteristics
20. Products or results

3. **Creating I:** Since LARC I can provide inventive solutions for many problems at this stage, examine each fact-bit for solutions. Compare fact-bits to other fact-bits. Record all creative ideas.

## LARC II

1. **Drawing:** Draw pictures of each word or concept you will use in the program.
   A. Draw specific pictures for specific terms (house, school) and symbolic pictures for symbolic terms (destruction, love).
   B. Draw several pictures from different angles, perspectives, etc., for each word.
2. **Smashing:** Use one of the four following lists — active, passive, simple, complex — to generate fact-bits from your terms.

*Passive*

*Simple*

1. Types
2. Steps
3. Parts
4. Causes
5. When
6. Why
7. How
8. Things connected with
9. Sight images of
10. Products or results

*Complex*

1. Types
2. Steps
3. Parts
4. Causes
5. Synonyms
6. Who
7. What
8. When
9. Where
10. Why
11. How
12. Things connected with
13. Sight images of
14. Hearing images of
15. Emotions
16. Opposite
17. Touching images of
18. Characteristics
19. Products or results
20. Modes of operation

*Active*

*Simple*

1. Abilities
2. Fear or threats
3. Goals and hopes
4. Strengths
5. Weaknesses
6. Types
7. Steps
8. Things connected with
9. Sight images of
10. Characteristics

*Complex*

1. Abilities
2. Fear or threats
3. Goals and hopes
4. Responsibilities
5. Interests
6. Likes
7. Dislikes
8. Strengths
9. Weaknesses
10. Types
11. Causes
12. Steps
13. How become
14. Who is
15. Where
16. When
17. Things connected with
18. Sight images of
19. Characteristics
20. Products or results

3. **Creating I:** Since LARC II can provide inventive solutions for many problems at this stage, examine each fact-bit to look for solutions. Compare fact-bits to other fact-bits. Record all creative ideas.
4. **Rearranging:** From the fact-bits the word lists have helped you produce, make Groups.
   A. Give a specific title to each symbol you create (e.g., "Group of Power," "Group of Seasons," etc.).
   B. Put an important fact-bit all by itself as a symbol.
5. **Creating II:** Generate new ideas.
   A. Examine each symbol and compare it to other symbols or fact-bits.
   B. Compare titles of the organizing symbols (Groups) to each other.
   C. Record all new ideas.

## LARC III

1. **Drawing:** Draw pictures of each word or concept you will use in the program.
   A. Draw specific pictures for specific terms (house, school) and symbolic pictures for symbolic terms (destruction, love).
   B. Draw several pictures from different angles, perspectives, etc., for each word.
2. **Smashing:** Use one of the four following lists — active, passive, simple, complex — to generate fact-bits from your terms.

*Passive*

*Simple*

1. Types
2. Steps
3. Parts
4. Causes
5. When
6. Why
7. How
8. Things connected with
9. Sight images of
10. Products or results

*Complex*

1. Types
2. Steps
3. Parts
4. Causes
5. Synonyms
6. Who
7. What
8. When
9. Where
10. Why
11. How
12. Things connected with
13. Sight images of
14. Hearing images of
15. Emotions
16. Opposite
17. Touching images of
18. Characteristics
19. Products or results
20. Modes of operation

*Active*

| *Simple* | *Complex* |
|---|---|
| 1. Abilities | 1. Abilities |
| 2. Fear or threats | 2. Fear or threats |
| 3. Goals and hopes | 3. Goals and hopes |
| 4. Strengths | 4. Responsibilities |
| 5. Weaknesses | 5. Interests |
| 6. Types | 6. Likes |
| 7. Steps | 7. Dislikes |
| 8. Things connected with | 8. Strengths |
| 9. Sight images of | 9. Weaknesses |
| 10. Characteristics | 10. Types |
| | 11. Causes |
| | 12. Steps |
| | 13. How become |
| | 14. Who is |
| | 15. Where |
| | 16. When |
| | 17. Things connected with |
| | 18. Sight images of |
| | 19. Characteristics |
| | 20. Products or results |

3. **Creating I:** Since LARC III can provide inventive solutions for many problems at this stage, examine each fact-bit for solutions. Compare fact-bits to other fact-bits. Record all creative ideas.
4. **Rearranging:** From the fact-bits the word lists have helped you produce make Groups, Pyramids, Chains, and Circles for each term.
   A. Give a specific title to each symbol you create (e.g.,"Pyramid of Power," "Cycle of Seasons," etc.).
   B. Put an important fact-bit all by itself as a symbol.
5. **Creating II:** Generate new ideas.
   A. Examine each symbol and compare it to other symbols or fact-bits.
   B. Compare titles of the organizing symbols (Groups, Pyramids, etc.) to each other.
   C. Record all creative ideas.

## *LARC IV*

1. **Stating the Problem:**
   A. Write sentences about the problem, being more specific each time.
   B. Underline the key words (or concepts) in your most specific sentences. These are the words and concepts you will pursue through LARC.
2. **Drawing:** Draw pictures of each word or concept you use.
   A. Draw specific pictures for specific terms (house, school) and symbolic pictures for symbolic terms (destruction, love).

B. Draw several pictures from different angles, perspectives, etc., for each word.

C. Find objects to look at, touch, etc., that remind you of the terms.

3. **Smashing:** Use one of the four following lists — active, passive, simple, complex — to generate fact-bits from your terms.

*Passive*

*Simple*

1. Types
2. Steps
3. Parts
4. Causes
5. When
6. Why
7. How
8. Things connected with
9. Sight images of
10. Products or results

*Complex*

1. Types
2. Steps
3. Parts
4. Causes
5. Synonyms
6. Who
7. What
8. When
9. Where
10. Why
11. How
12. Things connected with
13. Sight images of
14. Hearing images of
15. Emotions
16. Opposite
17. Touching images of
18. Characteristics
19. Products or results
20. Modes of operation

*Active*

*Simple*

1. Abilities
2. Fear or threats
3. Goals and hopes
4. Strengths
5. Weaknesses
6. Types
7. Steps
8. Things connected with
9. Sight images of
10. Characteristics

*Complex*

1. Abilities
2. Fear or threats
3. Goals and hopes
4. Responsibilities
5. Interests
6. Likes
7. Dislikes
8. Strengths
9. Weaknesses
10. Types
11. Causes
12. Steps
13. How become
14. Who is

*Complex*

15. Where
16. When
17. Things connected with
18. Sight images of
19. Characteristics
20. Products or results

4. **Creating I:** Since LARC IV can provide inventive solutions for many problems at this stage, examine each fact-bit for solutions. Compare fact-bits to other fact-bits. Record all creative ideas.
5. **Rearranging:** From the fact-bits the word lists have helped you produce make Groups, Pyramids, Chains, and Circles for each term.
   A. Give a specific title to each symbol you create (e.g., "Pyramid of Power," "Cycle of Seasons," etc.).
   B. Draw pictures beside the symbol, pictures that mean something (to *you*) about that symbol (Group, Pyramid, etc.).
   C. Put an important fact-bit all by itself as a symbol.
   D. Try to make Groups, Pyramids, etc., from the titles of your organizing symbols. This will produce larger concepts.
6. **Creating II:** Generate new ideas.
   A. Examine each symbol and compare it to other symbols or fact-bits.
   B. Compare titles of the organizing symbols (Groups, Pyramids, etc.) to each other.
   C. Draw the following Relationship Lines between fact-bits or organizing symbols to show pictorial relationships:

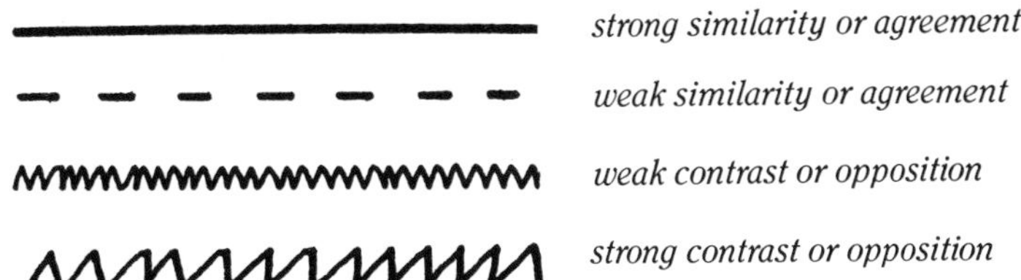


   D. Put each symbol on a 3″ x 5″ card to make it easier to match the symbols with each other.
   E. Record all creative ideas.

# part III
# LARC and Real Life

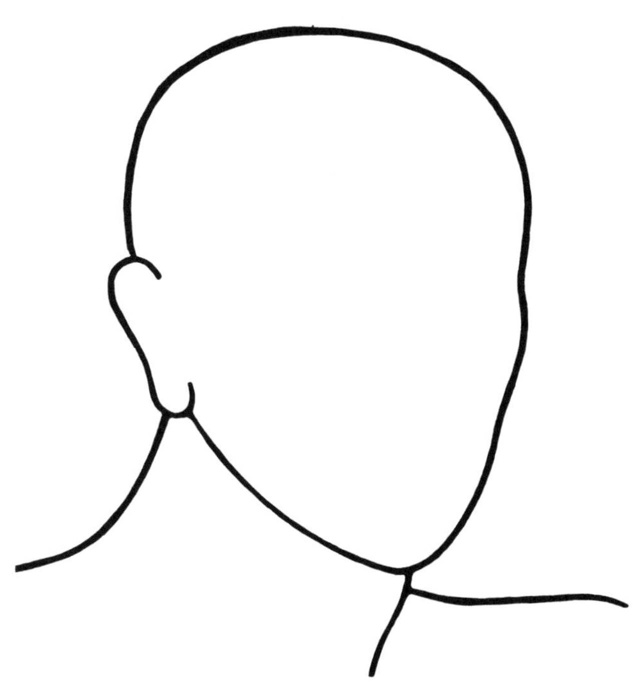

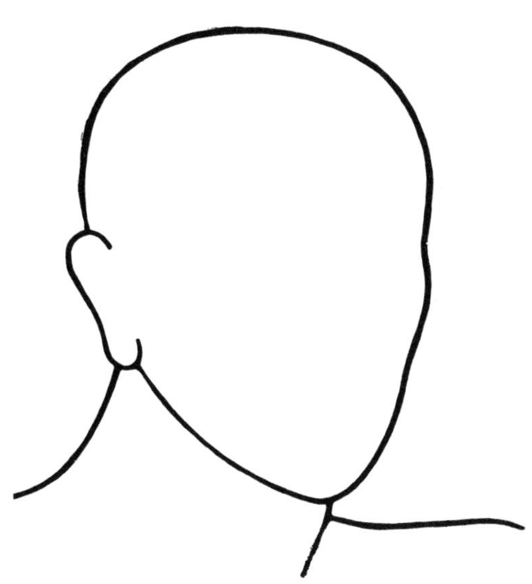

# 8 LARC and Real Life

Do you still doubt that LARC works on *real* problems? Do you find yourself asking, "But will it work for *me* ?" You can't be blamed for feeling this way, for you have yet to see LARC work on everyday problems. If it were possible, now would be the time to take one of *your* problems, to show that LARC does indeed work! There is no way to know what problems you would like to see illustrated, however. What we can show you, though, is how LARC helped answer other people's questions about the real world. And so three varied problems follow. First you will read about the difficulty, then the solution, and finally you'll see how LARC helped produce the creative response. (Although most problems can be solved by LARC I or II, the examples we've selected also use LARC III and IV. By reading these examples, not only will you see how LARC works on *real* problems, but you'll also get a better feel for how to apply the advanced versions.)

## Problems Solved

A college student working in campus publicity had already made two sports films on the college football team, doing them the usual way by showing big plays both on offense and defense, with background music and narrative describing the plays. But . . . he wasn't satisfied with them. And so he decided to try LARC for his third film. (In chapter 6 we discussed his efforts as an example of how to make a problem more specific.) His final statement of the problem was: how can I make a highlight film on my college football team that will be exciting and also informative and inspirational to potential recruits?

After running the words "film," "college football," "exciting," and "recruits" through LARC, the student decided to make the following film:

## *Football Highlight Film*

The film presented a week in the life of the college, leading up to the Saturday football game. There were quick cuts of the campus — student life, athletes attending class and practicing for the big game. His emphasis was on the athlete as student, to demonstrate the school's interest in academics as well as football. Interviews and candid shots revealed the school atmosphere and spirit, the winning tradition of the school. On Saturday morning, the stadium was first shown empty, then beginning to fill as students streamed across the campus to see the game. The excitement of the pre-game activities followed, then the game itself in which the home team was trailing until the very end of the fourth quarter. With big plays, the team came from behind to win — to the joy and camaraderie of athletes and students alike. In short, this production was a quantum leap over the student's earlier films. The student credited LARC for his new ideas.

How did LARC work for him? In a shortened version, here's what the student did with LARC.

Stating the Problem: How can I make a highlight *film* on my *college football* team that will be *exciting* and also informative and inspirational to potential *recruits*?

Using the underlined words as key terms, he smashed them, generating fact-bits. Then he produced symbols for each term: Groups, Pyramids, etc.; some of them are reproduced below.

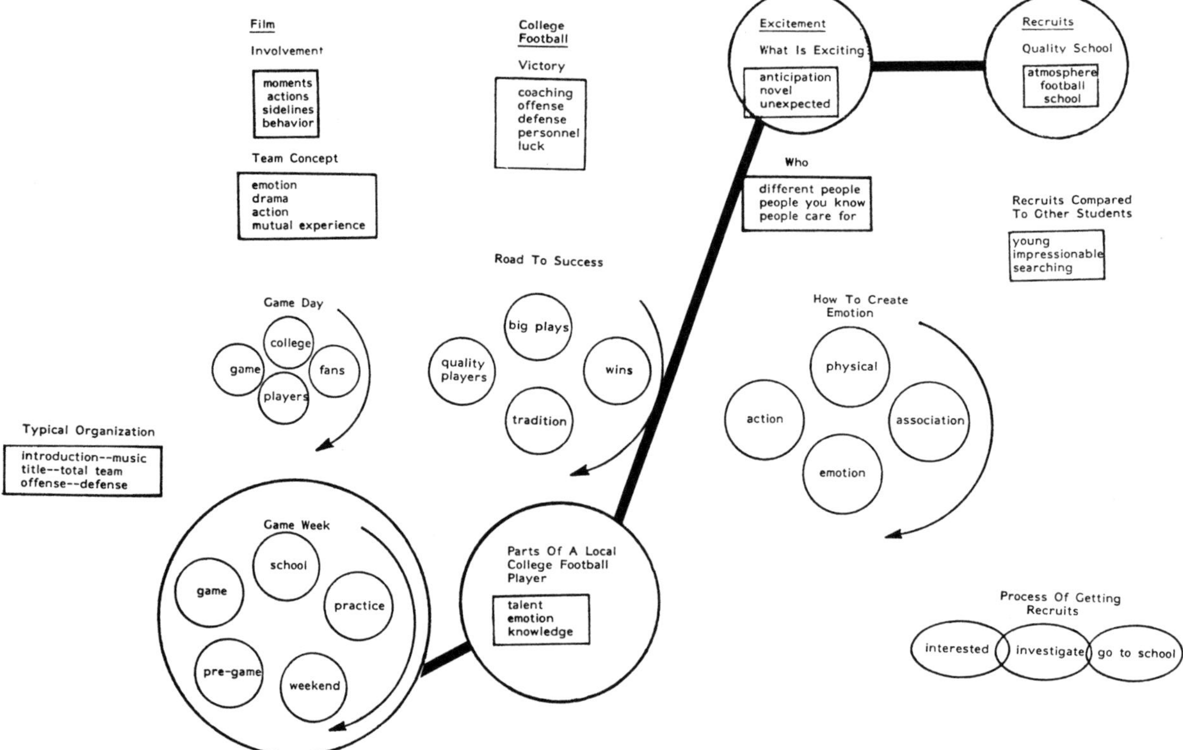

He decided to build his film around those symbols marked with the dark circles. Side by side, the four important symbols are as follows:

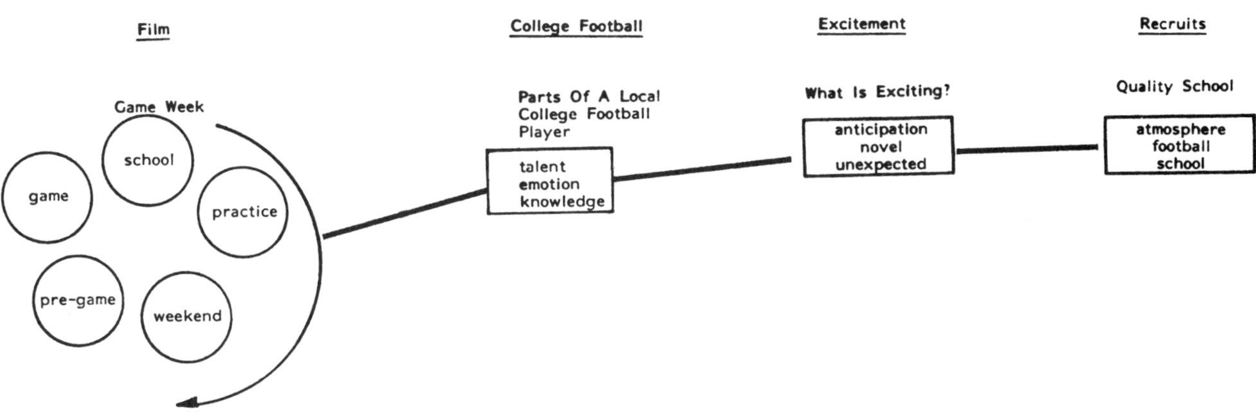


For the overall organization, he decided to use his Circle titled "Game Week," pumping into it the talent, emotion, and knowledge of the players as the week built toward the Saturday game. For anticipation, he used increasingly exciting music and narration as the week progressed and showed the weight room and athletes in classes – to demonstrate they had to learn things other than football. On game day, he began with footage of students surging into the stadium and followed this with clips of exciting plays as the team came from behind to win at the last minute. All this, he thought, would help with recruiting.

Let's take a second example. In this case, a man wished to design a co-ed game (a "pick-up" game to be played at picnics) that would be fun and fast-moving but that would not take any real skill or practice, or give men any advantage over women. After reworking his problem, he stated it as follows: "I want to invent a co-ed game that is fun and active, in which every player is the equal of every other player." By using LARC, he invented a game called Triple Ball. The rules of the game follow. You may even want to play it yourself. (Consider getting to play the game as this chapter's bonus – like the prize in the Cracker Jack box.)

## *Triple Ball*

**Teams:** *two teams;* minimum of two players each. Any number can play.

**Equipment:** *three balls* – whiffle ball, NeRF football, Frisbee. (The person who complains that a Frisbee is not a *ball* is the same type of person who grouches about Thales' having a stopwatch.)

Playing Field:

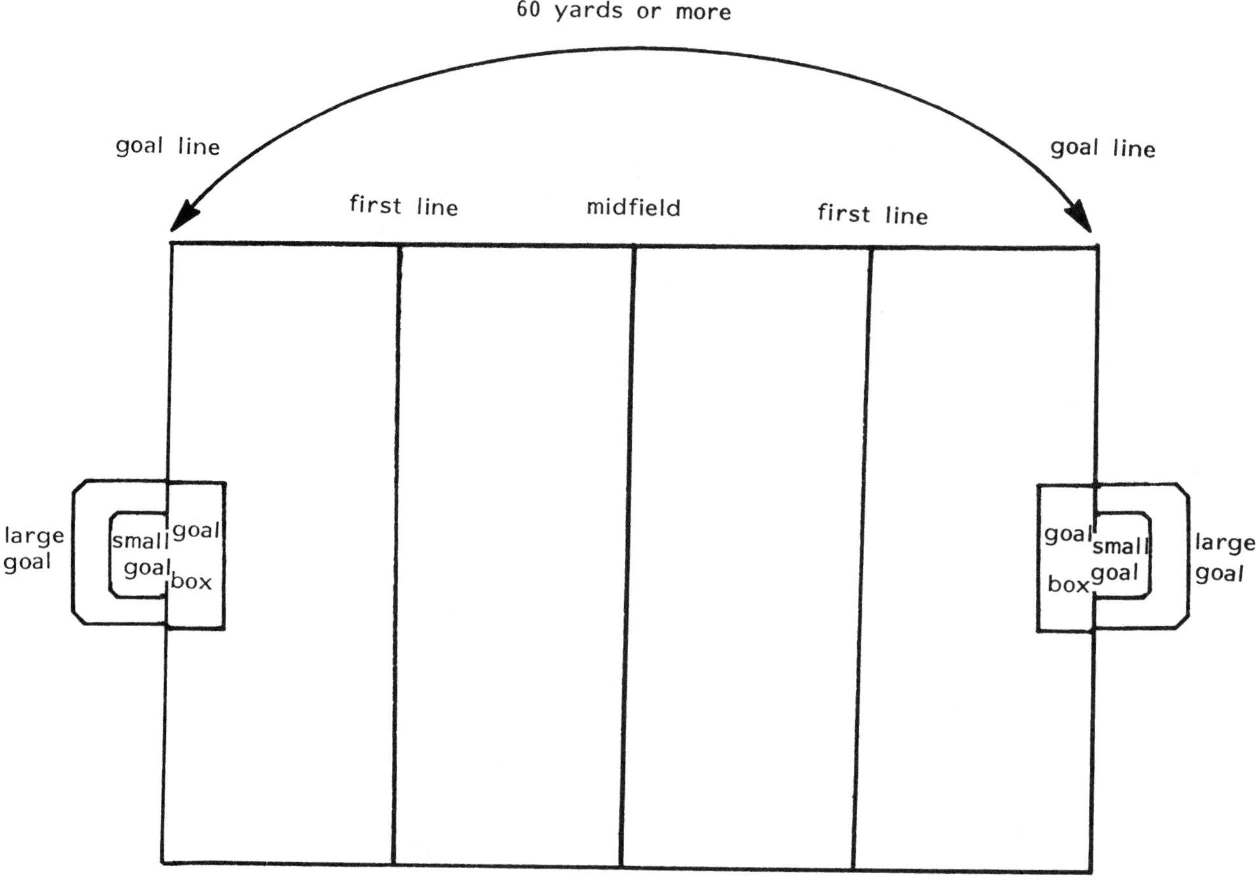


**General Rules:**

1. *Advancing the ball:* pass NeRF football (backward passes for boys, as in rugby; forward or backward passes for girls). Players may run with the ball after catching a pass. Pass Frisbee. Player may not run with Frisbee. Hit wiffle ball with bat only. The wiffle ball goes over to the other team, where it lands, unless there has been a score. No running or passing with this ball allowed.
2. *Change of possession:* ball changes possession if player knocks Frisbee or other balls out-of-bounds, if boy drops Frisbee or NeRF ball, or if either boy or girl is tagged (with one hand) while running with NeRF ball. Girls retain possession of all balls if they are caught while still rolling, but if a girl lets a ball stop, the other team gets possession.
3. *Switching balls:* at any time, a player with a ball may announce a change of balls. All play stops. Player goes to sideline to get another ball, then returns to spot where announcement was made and resumes play with new ball.
4. *General defense:* no direct physical contact is allowed.

Scoring:

1. *Whiffle:* score *one point* if the whiffle is hit in the air over opponents' goal line. The same team member may score whiffles until goal is missed or defense stops ball. Boys may attempt whiffle only from midfield zone. Girls may attempt whiffle from offensive zone (inside opponents' first line). If boys catch ball before it hits ground, no score is made; ball changes teams. If girls catch ball on the roll there is no score and the ball changes teams, but girls cannot "save" balls that have been touched and dropped by another defender. If players are stopped by defenders, the defenders have choice of ball when play resumes. Ball changes begin at team's own first line.
2. *Frisbee:* a Frisbee thrown through a goal scores *three points.* Boys throw through small goal. Girls throw through large goal. Both girls and boys throw from outside goal box. Throws must pass goal less than six feet in air. Boys must pass goal in the air; girls may roll Frisbee over goal. Only one player may defend goal box (by knocking Frisbee down, catching it, etc.). After successful or unsuccessful attempt at goal, other team takes possession from spot where Frisbee lands. They may play it from where they pick it up. If opponent has scored, they may have choice of any ball, starting at their first line.
   *Special rule on taking shots with Frisbee:* (1) unannounced shot—player just shoots; all defenders defend as best they can; (2) announced shot—player announces he or she is going to shoot. One defender (only one) stands in goal box to defend before the shot. Shooter takes shot.
3. *NeRF:* a NeRF scores *two points.* To score a NeRF, a player must run through the opposing team's goal area with the NeRF ball (small goal, boys; large goal, girls) without being touched by an opponent.

End of Game: Play continues until teams reach agreed-upon score, or for an agreed-upon time limit.

That's the game, and an imaginative one it is. Here is how the person used LARC to develop it. He began by deciding what he wanted to invent.

> *Stating the Problem:* "I want to invent a *co-ed game* that is fun and active, in which every player is *equal* to every other player.

On looking over these concepts, he decided that the word "game" was too broad and broke it down into "field," "offense," and "defense" by referring to a few Smashing questions ("parts" and "steps" of a game). He decided to leave out "active," but to keep it in the back of his mind. Then he converted co-ed game into the words "equality of sexes" since he really wanted a game in which women would be equal to men. Now he had his words: field, offense, defense, and equality of sexes. This completed the step, Stating the Problem.

Next he broke down these four concepts using the Smashing questions to generate fact-bits for each word. After Creating I, he arranged fact-bits into Groups, Pyramids, etc., a few of which are listed below.

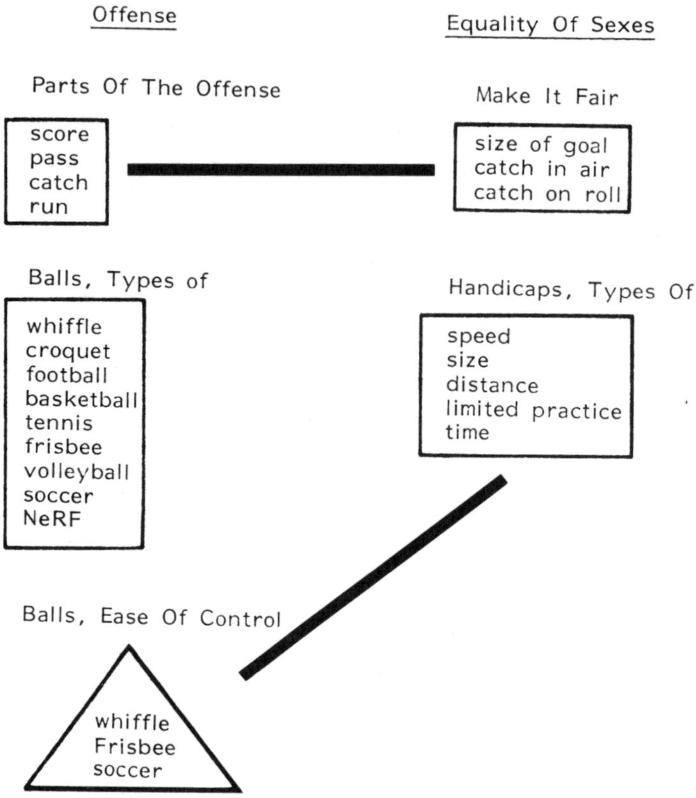


After drawing two strong-similarity Relationship Lines, he made some decisions. He wanted action so he discarded the croquet ball as too slow. Since men might have practiced more with a basketball and regular football, these balls were discarded as well. He found a Circle (below) around which to build the game.

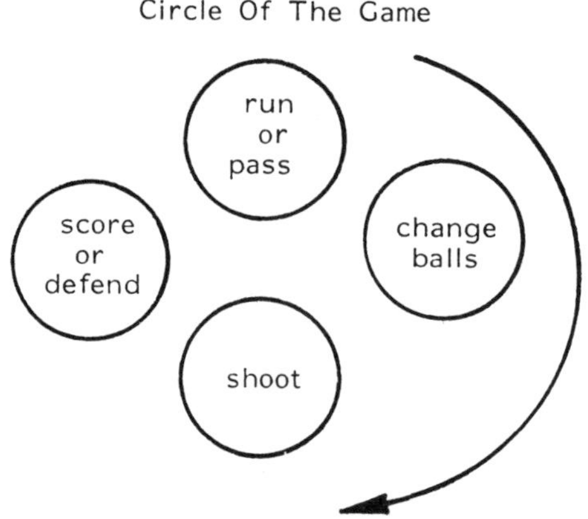


Other parts of LARC were important (fact-bit comparison in Creating I, etc.), but you can see how much of the game was generated by looking at the symbols given.

In our third example, LARC helped a university student write a paper for a class in graduate school. (You don't need to understand the details of the following example in order to see how LARC helped.) The student's paper was about similarities between "behaviorism" (man functions like a machine) and "humanism" (man has free will and controls his own behavior). This was a difficult undertaking because these two ideas of human behavior are generally thought to be opposing positions. The following Group and Pyramid made all the difference to his paper:

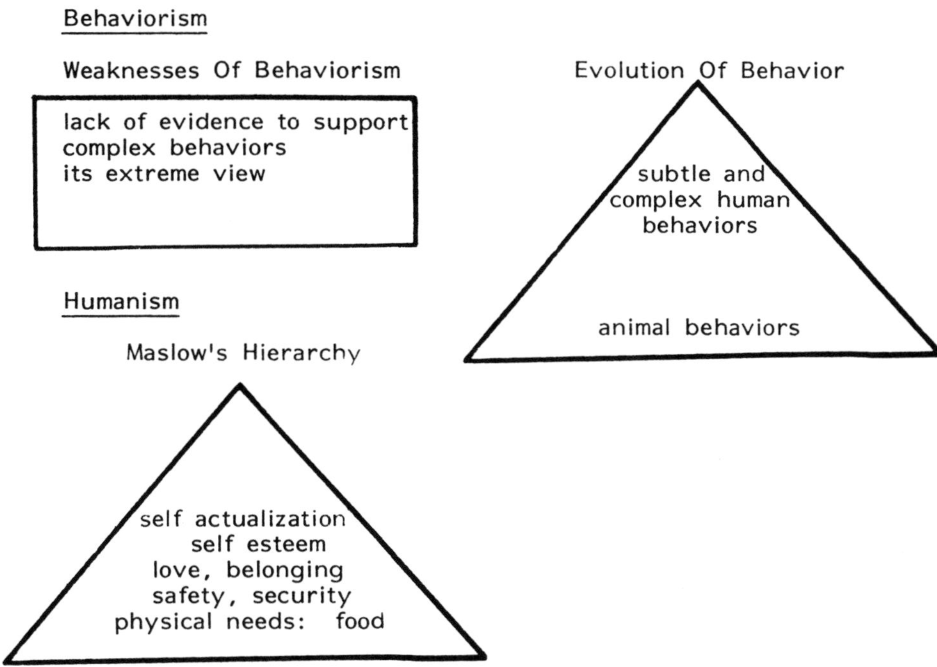


Again, it is important not that you understand what is at issue here, but that you see the process. After looking at the organizing symbols above, the student was struck by the similarity of *shapes* between his "Evolution of Behavior" Pyramid and the "Maslow's Hierarchy" Pyramid. This structural similarity led him to carefully examine fact-bits within each Pyramid to see if there was any connection. While not finding any direct relation among the terms, he did make an intriguing observation that applied to each theory (gained, in part, from the Group titled "Weaknesses of Behaviorism"): "Both behaviorism and humanism can find some pretty solid proof for their simple assertions. That is, the behaviorist can readily give examples of how animal behaviors are conditioned, while the humanists find it easy to show how all humans have physical needs. However, for both schools, there is a notable absence of tangible proof for their more extreme assertions. The behaviorists have trouble showing how all complex human behaviors can be reduced to reinforcement, and the humanists would be pressed to give concrete evidence of self actualization." His professors were pleased by this insight in his paper; the student credited LARC for helping him generate that idea.

You have now been shown three practical problems that LARC helped to solve: the film, the game, and the graduate paper. Of course, these solutions were not relevant to you — only *your* problems would be.

By this time, your eyes may be clouding over as you consider the number of times you must apply LARC to your problems. But, of course, you wouldn't have to use it for most of your difficulties. Problems that fit the left brain's preset patterns are solved all the time without special help. Try LARC only for those questions that take a creative solution. This is the specialty of LARC — prompting the right-left brain switching so crucial in the production of new ideas. Again, the speculation is that some people have learned, by accident, to do this switching automatically, quickly. (And even these "naturally creative" few will find that LARC will enhance their inventiveness.) Now the rest of us also have the chance to stimulate the same creative left-right brain interaction (only more slowly) by using LARC.

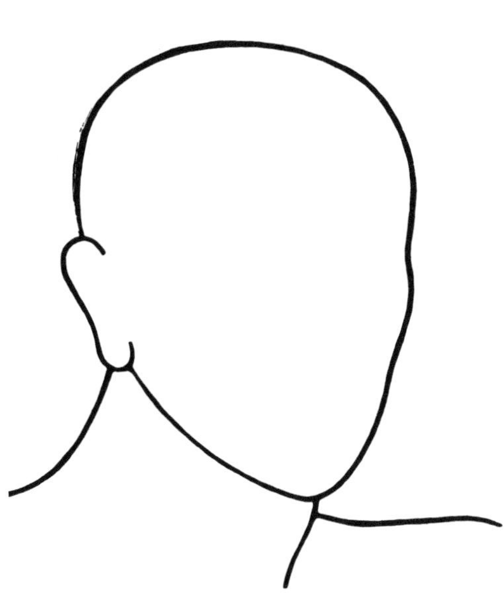

# 9 Theory into Practice

No matter how others have used LARC, what is important is that you use it to solve your own nagging, creativity problems. Difficulties requiring an inventive solution could be . . . anything . . . but what?

Because, even after learning LARC, some people still seem to be puzzled about just how to use LARC in their own lives, this chapter suggests more situations in which LARC can be applied. (In fact, for many of these problems, LARC *has* been helpful to someone in the *real world.*) Again, the problems mentioned here — broad as they are — may not be identical to those *you* would like to examine. It is our hope, though, that with enough examples you will see something that parallels a difficulty you are having, one for which LARC can help you find the *perfect answer.*

## Uses of LARC

### The Creative Endeavor — Art and Writing

Do you have to come up with a topic for a term paper? Do you want to paint a picture or write a poem? We think (we have done this ourselves) that LARC is excellent for those projects that, by definition, are creative. Authors in search of "flesh and blood" characters could use LARC to "see" their characters from all sides. LARC could be used for "plots" (for example, run "murder" through to get new angles on it). By using LARC, artists wishing to explore such themes as youth, love, patriotism etc. may get useful ideas about how to represent these abstract concepts.

## Job Choice

Uncertain about what job to take? Confused? To the rescue comes LARC! One man approached a job search the following way. First, he ran his "goals" through LARC to clarify what he wanted out of life. Then he examined each of three possible "jobs" with LARC. Comparing the insights LARC gave him (fact-bits from goals and from each of the three jobs), he made a job choice about which he felt more certain and which, to date, has proved a good one.

## Problems on the Job — Productivity

We (our bosses?) are all concerned about doing a better job at work and being more productive. Yet, we sometimes find ourselves "stuck" with a problem for which the solution seems elusive. Using LARC, there is hope. In the first place, most people know much technical information about their jobs, and as Graham Wallas put it, have already passed the Preparation stage of the creative process. What they really need is to break up old patterns. So, to see things differently, they can plug in LARC to find key terms connected with the problem, then smash these terms into fact-bits, and rearrange these fact-bit fragments.

One hypothetical use of LARC for such a "work" problem is trying to solve a weakness in office communications by some kind of reorganization. Running the terms "office," "communication," and "arrangements" through LARC might spark new concepts of how the office could be structured for better communication.

## Problems with Relationships

Have a problem with a co-worker, neighbor, relative? Examining the key factors or terms of this difficult interpersonal relationship may release information — and in combinations you may not have considered — that will surprise you. If the problem is the personality of another person, you might explore *yourself*, to see more precisely what *you* are like (your goals, ideas, interests, etc.), and then process the other person. LARC can help you gain fresh angles for the solution of problems with someone else by showing you how you are similar or dissimilar to others.

## The Perfect Date

When trying to impress that "certain someone," who *hasn't* wished to take her (him?) on a perfect date? (Even more important may be finding the answer to the question, "How can I keep this date from turning into a *disaster*?" (One man confessed to us that he had rarely had a date in high school without suffering the greatest apprehension. Oh, *think* how his anxiety might have been alleviated if only he had had LARC to help him! But . . . it's not too late for *you*. You might try, for instance, the term "*date*" with LARC. Another man did this. To answer the Smashing question "sight images of," he wrote: a romantic scene by a river in the woods. Combining this with the fact-bit "wine" from "parts" of a date and the fact-bit "eating out" from "types" of a date, he thought of having a picnic in a

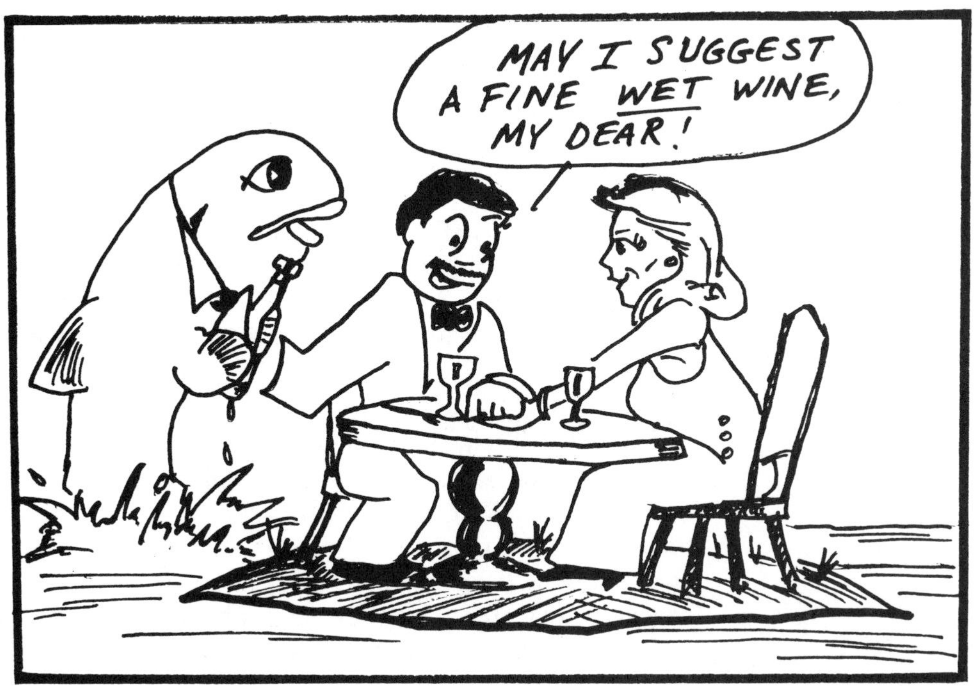


wooded area by a brook and even went to the spot early to place a bottle of wine in the stream. He said his date was impressed when, at the right time, he went to the brook to retrieve the properly chilled bottle. The rest, as they say, is history, which leads us to . . .

## *Planning a Wedding*

For almost everyone, a wedding is . . . special. A person might approach this goal by exploring the term "wedding" to discover just what meanings this experience has that could be included in the actual event. For instance, if the couple met on a tennis court (they could have gotten the fact-bit "tennis" from smashing "steps" of a wedding), they might include the theme of tennis in their wedding. One couple did this; along with rice, friends tossed tennis balls at them following the ceremony. In the same vein, Sarah Ferguson (her husband, Prince Andrew, a helicopter pilot with the British navy) made anchors and waves part of her wedding gown. (Could *they* have been using LARC?)

## *The "Ideal" Vacation*

For many, vacations are not just "nice" but essential, and we wish to get the most out of them. Often, however, when a couple (Joe and Sally) are planning a vacation, they disagree on what would be the best holiday. Both Joe and Sally could run the word "vacation" through LARC, and discover similarities and differences in their respective ideas of the perfect holiday. Comparing these ideas may allow them to decide just where they wish to go, what location should be avoided, etc. Used in this way, LARC could help them decide on a single vacation that would be "perfect" for each of them.

## *The "Dream" House*

What better way to think of features for the "dream house" than with a system that produces the kinds of creative visions often associated with *dreams*? "House" would be a term to try with LARC. Perhaps terms like "luxurious" (if money is no object) or "comfortable" (if money *is* an object?) might also be used.

## *Self-Understanding or Self Goals*

Would you like an example of something more abstract for which LARC might be of help? One thing all of us are seeking is self-understanding. Use LARC for *yourself.* Doing that, you may learn something important about yourself, of which you may have been only marginally aware. In the same vein, one person explored "goals" with LARC to help her clarify what was most important to her and to decide what activities she should pursue to make these goals become realities.

## *Creativity: A Final Word*

Creativity is not only an "art" but also a skill, one that can be taught to anyone. Furthermore, studies have shown that LARC, designed as it is to trigger both left- and right-brain input, is an excellent method for learning this skill; a person practicing with LARC finds creative ideas coming more quickly. And finally, coupling inventive insights with the courage to use them in the real world is creativity maximized.

Creative thought followed by creative action — this is a formula that breeds success in problem-solving, in work, in relationships, and in life!